Psychosis and Personality Disorders

Paola Rocca • Silvio Bellino
Editors

Psychosis and Personality Disorders

Unmet Needs in Early Diagnosis and Treatment

Springer

Editors
Paola Rocca
Department of Neuroscience
University of Turin
Turin, Italy

Silvio Bellino
Department of Neuroscience
University of Turin
Turin, Italy

ISBN 978-3-031-09057-8 ISBN 978-3-031-09058-5 (eBook)
https://doi.org/10.1007/978-3-031-09058-5

This Springer imprint is published by the registered company Springer Nature Switzerland AG
The registered company address is: Gewerbestrasse 11, 6330 Cham, Switzerland

Contents

1 **Trajectories Toward Bipolar Disorder or Schizophrenia in FEP and High-Risk Mental State** 1
Cecilia Riccardi, Cristiana Montemagni, Silvio Bellino, Paola Bozzatello, and Paola Rocca

2 **New Strategies to Improve Cognitive Symptom Domain in the Treatment of Schizophrenia** 19
Stefano Barlati, Cassandra Ariu, Andrea Garozzo, and Antonio Vita

3 **Psychotic Disorders and Substance Abuse Comorbidity: Characteristics and Treatment** 57
Kirsten Catthoor and Geert Dom

4 **Recovery from Psychosis: Definition, Paradoxes, and Clinical Implications** 75
Paul H. Lysaker

5 **Cluster A Personality Disorders and Potential for Early Intervention in Psychosis: Challenges and Opportunities** 87
Saeed Farooq and Muhammad Ayub

6 **Risk Factors of Early Onset of Borderline Personality Disorder: A Conceptual Model** 107
Silvio Bellino, Marco Bosia, Cristiana Montemagni, Paola Rocca, and Paola Bozzatello

7 **Clinical Evaluation and Intervention of Emerging Psychosis: A Mentalization-Informed Perspective** 125
Martin Debbané, George Salaminios, Jonas Weijers, Peter Fonagy, Eduardo Fonseca-Pedrero, and Marco Armando

8 **Personality Disorders and Suicidality** 145
Marco Sarchiapone and Patrizia Zeppegno

Trajectories Toward Bipolar Disorder or Schizophrenia in FEP and High-Risk Mental State

1

Cecilia Riccardi, Cristiana Montemagni, Silvio Bellino, Paola Bozzatello, and Paola Rocca

1.1 Introduction

Considering cognitive and functional impairment, inadequate clinical response and relapsing course, schizophrenia (SCZ) and bipolar disorder (BPD) are two of the most relevant mental disorders [1, 2]. Increasing evidences are pointing out significant clinical, cognitive, and genetic overlap between these two disorders [3] suggesting the existence of a wider category of "psychosis spectrum" [4]. Clinically, it can be hard to differentiate early phases of SCZ and BPD, which often present common characteristics, especially when psychotic symptoms are prevalent in BPD.

Comprehensive early intervention services are the key to improve a range of outcomes, including global functioning, compared to usual care [5, 6]. Unfortunately, many of these specialized programs focus mainly on subjects thought to have a psychotic-spectrum diagnosis, excluding patients whose initial diagnosis was on the affective spectrum [7, 8]. Nevertheless, diagnostic shifts in first episode psychosis (FEP) are frequent, with shifts from affective to non-affective diagnoses, and vice versa [9]. Therefore, it is easy to understand that diagnostic validity is a crucial issue with an increasing focus on FEP field research. In 2016, Fusar-Poli and colleagues published a large meta-analysis identifying 42 studies for a total of 14,484 patients with FEP and found out that SCZ, BPD with psychosis, depression with psychosis and schizoaffective disorder have a relatively high diagnostic stability, all above 70% (with SCZ and BPD 90%), instead schizophreniform disorder and psychosis not otherwise specified are a lot more unstable [10]. More recently, Cawkwell et al. [11] conducted a retrospective chart review on diagnostic stability over a 2 years follow-up, their sample was made of 96 patients, aged between 18 and 30 years,

C. Riccardi · C. Montemagni · S. Bellino · P. Bozzatello · P. Rocca (✉)
Department of Neuroscience, University of Turin, Turin, Italy
e-mail: cecilia.riccardi@unito.it; cristiana.montemagni@unito.it; silvio.bellino@unito.it; paola.bozzatello@unito.it; paola.rocca@unito.it

P. Rocca, S. Bellino (eds.), *Psychosis and Personality Disorders*,
https://doi.org/10.1007/978-3-031-09058-5_1

with FEP who maintained engagement for at least 24 months. Consistently with previous results, they confirmed a generally high rate of stability, all above 80%, in SCZ and BPD diagnoses [11].

A frequent cause of diagnostic uncertainty is that these patients often present simultaneous manifestations of psychotic, manic and disorganized cluster symptoms, especially at early stages. During FEP the validity of the diagnosis can be threatened by the overlap of nonspecific symptoms. Some researchers argue that there was, particularly in the past, a widespread tendency to diagnose SCZ whenever psychotic symptoms are present [12].

In this chapter, we aim to better understand what is known in literature about FEP's trajectory toward SCZ or BPD diagnosis, in order to establish whether there are indicators in the early stages of disease that could be used to improve targeted therapy and to reduce the significant burden of these serious mental illnesses.

The outcome of FEP is still very variable, ranging from early recovery to antipsychotic treatment resistance; naturalistic follow-up studies have been made and found different outcomes [13]. Interestingly, individuals with an initial diagnosis of non-affective psychosis seem to experience a worse clinical course and outcome [13].

For clinicians, the possibility to predict the trajectory of these patients and their diagnoses would be highly valuable to select the most appropriate therapy and to tailor psychosocial and psychoeducational treatments, in fact, treatment options can be substantially different and might impact morbidity and mortality. Nowadays, the challenge in treating FEP patients is to predict these different trajectories [14]. Major efforts have been made to identify diagnosis-specific biomarkers that can help differentiate between SCZ and BPD. To our knowledge, this challenge represents an important current unmet need. To try to find an answer we gathered evidences present in modern literature about FEP and we selected four macro-areas of interest to deepen: differences and overlaps in genetics, cognition, neuroimaging, and prodrome/clinical features of FEP patients considering their later diagnoses.

1.2 Genetics

Over the past two decades, researchers have placed increasing attention on the study of genetic alterations in psychiatric disorders. Several important studies have reported alterations in gene products or genes shared by SCZ and BPD [15–17]. In fact, many laboratories, guided by the hypothesis of genetic overlap in the main psychotic disorders, have studied and documented common genetic variants [15, 16, 18] taking into account the existence of a common underlying pathogenic mechanism.

In 2005, Walss-Bass and colleagues used a phenotype characterized by manic symptoms to identify an overlap of genetic loci in SCZ and BPD patients. Subsequently, other studies have deepened overlaps among autism disorder spectrum, SCZ, and BPD [19, 20].

An important example is represented by AKT1, a known protein involved in signaling networks with a pivotal role in neurodevelopment: in early 2000 its gene variants have been associated with SCZ [21, 22] and BPD [23].

Karege et al. [24] confirmed that there is a genetic overlap between SCZ and BPD and that AKT1 has a crucial role on it. Using a sample of 364 patients suffering from SCZ, BPD, or schizoaffective disorder and 165 healthy controls (HC), they demonstrated that AKT1 gene variants were associated separately with the symptoms involved in the diagnosis of SCZ and BPD; specific variants were commonly associated with a mood disorder, psychosis, and their various combinations. Data suggested that specific alleles are overrepresented in patients and that there is a correspondence between specific phenotypes and allelic variants. However, considering the possible interplay with environmental factors and the relatively small size of the sample, these findings needed further confirmation. Indeed, more recent genetic studies [25, 26] have expressed doubts about the reliability of the genes so far associated with SCZ. Farrell et al. [25] conducted a review about candidate genes for SCZ that were prominent in the literature and highlighted the lack of replicable results, whereas Johnson et al. [26] argued that variants in the most-studied candidate genes were no more associated with SCZ than variants in control sets of noncandidate genes. According to their study, a small subset of candidate genes did appear to be significantly associated with SCZ, but these genes were not particularly noteworthy considering a large number of more strongly associated noncandidate genes.

To deepen this topic researchers are now focusing on the potential value of the genome-wide association (GWA) studies, whole genome sequencing studies, and specific damaging alternative forms identified with GWA to predict the outcomes of FEP. GWA studies have become very accurate in estimating polygenic risk score (PRS), a weighted sum of trait-associated alleles. PRS has two related but distinct applications; first, testing for association between the score and its trait in the replication sample can determine whether associated markers reside within those contributing to the score. Second and perhaps more usefully, the PRS can be used to predict individual trait values or risks of disease [27], potentially becoming a predictor of treatment response and long-term outcomes in specific diseases. The first successful application of PRS analysis to GWA data was in SCZ [28]. It was shown that a large mass, up to half, of all markers in one GWA could be jointly associated with disease in a second sample, implying a polygenic component to disease risk that justified larger study sizes [29]. Furthermore, markers from SCZ GWA studies could together be associated with BPD, and vice versa, establishing a common polygenic basis for those conditions [30]. Interestingly, patients with BPD and high SCZ PRS are more likely to show mood incongruent psychotic symptoms [31]. In turn, patients with SCZ and BPD PRS are more likely to have severe manic symptoms. Moreover, BPD PRS is associated with psychotic symptoms in BPD patients [32].

The great potential of a PRS is that it represents a stable trait feature. Therefore, it is necessary to deepen the genetic line of research as it could redefine the current conception of psychiatric categories, making an improvement in the clinical management of these patients and in the choice of therapeutic strategies.

1.3 Cognitive Impairment

Cognitive impairment is one of the most relevant dimensions across different psychiatric disorders [33]. In SCZ and BPD, it has massive implications for long-term functional outcomes, such as lower rates of employment, difficulties in living independently, and in building stable relationships [34]. There is a very substantial literature on the relation between cognitive impairment and functional outcome in SCZ. According to the World Psychiatry Association, the current question is no longer whether but how cognition is related to functional outcome. Considering the highly complex nature of community functioning in SCZ or any other condition, it is clear that many of the observed relationships between cognition and community integration involve mediating variables.

Moreover, the identification of such key mediators is very important, because it can suggest specific therapeutic targets [35]. Several cognitive patterns have been investigated in the last decade; the robust and reliable nature of these deficits has led researchers to deepen the analysis on timing and profile of impairments, as this may clarify different neurodevelopmental patterns in individuals who experience psychosis [36].

Several studies found that the difference between SCZ and BPD cognitive patterns seems to be quantitative rather than qualitative. Indeed, SCZ patients appear to be quantitatively more affected [37, 38]. Cuesta et al. [39] and Lewandowski et al. [40] suggested that premorbid cognitive impairment may be the key to distinguish future SCZ or BPD evolution. Cuesta et al.'s aims were to examine the pattern and magnitude of cognitive impairment in FEP patients, the profile of impairment across psychosis subtypes and the associations with premorbid adjustment. To do so, they considered a sample of 266 FEP patients and 225 HC that were assessed in the PEPsCog study, as part of the PEPs study. Patients were grouped into three categories: SCZ spectrum, affective spectrum (which included BPD I and II and depressive episodes with psychotic symptoms), and other psychoses (OP). Assessments were made on five occasions: at recruitment, at 2 months, at 6 months, at 1 year, and at 2 years. Controls were only assessed at recruitment and at 2 years. The patients' cognitive assessments were performed at the 2-month visit to ensure their clinical stability. According to their results, a slight to moderate cognitive impairment was found in the entire patient group compared to controls. Moreover, the affective group outperformed the SCZ and OP groups in executive function, showed higher premorbid IQ than both groups and also less global cognitive impairment than the SCZ group. A review by Lewandowski et al. [41] focused on neuropsychological functioning in patients with SCZ, BPD, and related disorders before and after illness onset. They considered neurocognitive dysfunction as a core feature of all psychotic illnesses and traced its evolution from premorbid and prodromal states to the emergence of overt psychosis and into chronic illness in patients with SCZ and

BPD. Results showed that SCZ patients exhibit dysfunction before the illness's onset. Retrospective studies suggest that, on average, general intelligence is lower in individuals who later develop SCZ, and specific neurocognitive domains may be affected. This impairment appears pronounced in the prodrome and early years after diagnosis, then settles into a stable pattern. Conversely, patients with BPD generally exhibit typical cognitive development premorbidly, but demonstrate deficits after first episode that are amplified with worsening symptoms and exacerbations. After illness onset, both disorders appear to be associated with cognitive impairment, but in SCZ it seems to be more severe [42].

When coming to genetic high risk for affective disorder individuals, adolescents seem to exhibit similar neurocognitive deficits compared to young adults at risk for SCZ [43]. Few studies have concentrated on adolescents and young adults at genetic risk for SCZ and BPD, considering "at genetic risk" the offspring of patients. Children and siblings of SCZ and BPD patients have been compared to children and siblings of HC. Subjects of the high-risk SCZ (HRSCZ) group were significantly impaired on neurocognitive functioning, particularly in verbal ability, visual spatial functions, and working memory; subjects high-risk for BPD (HRBD) performed slightly better than HRSCZ but overall worse than controls [44]. Interestingly, Maziade et al. [45] compared similar subjects' samples with an extensive neurocognitive battery and found no difference in Wisconsin Card Sorting Test (WCST) total errors between HRSCZ and controls, but confirmed an overall decrease in cognitive functioning, particularly evident in memory tasks. The overlapping impairments in subjects with HRSCZ and HRBD probably reflect the existing overlapping in gene susceptibility, moreover, it seems reasonable that the common characteristics showed by the two major diseases in adulthood would originate in childhood. Unfortunately, even if cognitive differences between HRSCZ and HRBD exist, these would not probably be specific enough to orient toward SCZ or BPD evolution in at-risk subjects [45].

As regards specific cognitive domains, a systematic review highlighted the presence of a premorbid IQ impairment in young people who subsequently developed SCZ [46], instead the presence of this impairment is controversial in BPD. It is necessary to consider that few studies have investigated premorbid cognitive deficits in BPD patients, and the findings are equivocal. Sheffield and colleagues conducted a meta-analysis in 2018 and found a fallacy of many studies [40, 47–49] in finding evidence of significant premorbid cognitive impairments or premorbid IQ deficits among children and adolescents who subsequently developed BPD [50–52]. Furthermore, there is some evidence that higher cognitive functioning is associated with the development of BPD [42, 53–56]. According to Koenen et al. [57], a higher IQ score in childhood is significantly associated with mania. A significant limitation of the existing literature is the lack of studies comparing BPD with and without psychotic features on premorbid cognitive functioning [36]. In fact, the fewer studies that deepened it have revealed that the presence of psychotic features may worsen IQ deficits [58] and that patients with early onset of BPD with psychotic features showed IQ deficits [59]. It is important to highlight that these impairments are generally less severe than those found in premorbid SCZ [58, 60,

61]. Cognitive reserve could become a valid focus for clinical interventions to prevent cognitive and functional deficits. A study conducted on 266 FEP patients and 225 HC found a correlation between poor premorbid adjustment to a generalized cognitive impairment and low premorbid intellectual reserve [39]. On the contrary, a high cognitive reserve predicts a better psychosocial and cognitive outcome in BPD [62–64].

Interestingly, it also appears that cognitive deficit in FEP might be associated with the presence of negative symptoms. Specifically, the working memory cognitive domain seems significantly related to negative psychotic symptoms and to psychosocial functioning [65]. Cognitive deficits and negative symptoms share many features, such as a similar type of onset and course, and they are both associated with functional outcomes [66]. It appears that patients with FEP, which later develop an affective psychosis (bipolar, schizoaffective, depression with psychosis), have better performance in executive functions and less negative symptoms compared with patients that develop non-affective psychosis. After 2 years of follow-up, the non-affective group still has more negative symptoms, but no differences can be found in neuropsychological performance between the two groups [4]. The framework of these findings is a 2-year follow-up study conducted by the PEPS group on a total of 335 patients with FEP and 253 HC. Five assessments were made (baseline, 2 months, 6 months, 1 year, and 2 years). Torrent and colleagues included in their study 192 FEP patients who completed the follow-up at 2 years and who had, additionally, the functional assessment measure collected. Of these 192 FEP patients, 142 were non-affective and 50 affective. The aim was to assess any difference (clinical, functional, or neuropsychological) between non-affective and affective psychoses, in order to find predictors of psychosocial functioning. Interestingly, they also found that, in the whole sample, lower performance in verbal fluency tasks at baseline predicted a poor functional outcome; phonological verbal fluency requires the generation of a list of words from a letter indicated by investigator, this task involves high ability on executive functions. The key role of verbal fluency as a predictor of poor outcome is in line with current literature. It should be noticed that this study has some limitations: first, the study participants maintained their usual treatment and drug treatment was not controlled, this could have limited the evaluation of some variables. Second, the patient groups were not homogeneous, the non-affective FEP group was much larger than the affective FEP group. Verbal fluency was also the focus of Costafreda et al. [67] work. Using functional magnetic resonance imaging (fMRI) scans on subjects (SCZ, BPD, and HC) performing a phonological verbal fluency task, they found greater activation in SCZ patients, suggesting that verbal fluency could be a stronger diagnostic marker for SCZ than for BPD. This finding could represent a step forward in the identification and development of diagnostic biomarkers based on neural features, specific to each disorder. These findings should be replicated in future studies in patients who are medication-free in order to exclude potentially confounding effects. Interestingly, recent literature suggests that verbal fluency deficit occurs at an early stage of illness and remains stable in time. In fact, no correlation was found between verbal fluency and illness duration [68].

1.4 Neuroimaging

Another line of research is represented by neuroimaging. Consolidated evidence from the literature has highlighted the brain areas involved in major psychiatric disorders: BPD is characterized by reductions in prefrontal and paralimbic regions (anterior cingulate cortex and insula); SCZ is associated to diffuse frontotemporal gray matter reductions and ventricular enlargement [69, 70]. Interestingly, these deficits occur in early phases of psychosis, but with slight differences between affective (A-FEP) and non-affective FEP (NA-FEP): A-FEP patients show a significant reduction in total intracranial and white matter volumes [71], while NA-FEP shows ventricular enlargement and whole brain and hippocampal volumes [72, 73].

A multicenter cross-sectional case control brain magnetic resonance imaging (MRI) study suggests that age at FEP modulates the structural brain abnormalities in a nonlinear and diagnosis-dependent manner [74]. This study was conducted on 196 patients with FEP and 157 HC, and explored the relationship between age at scan and volume and thickness measurements, differentiating between patients with SCZ spectrum disorders, A-FEP, and HC. Subjects with early onset of SCZ (before 15–20 years) showed significant volume and thickness deficits in frontal lobe, volume deficits in temporal lobe, and volume enlargements in the ventricular system and basal ganglia. Subjects with early A-FEP (18–20 years) had smaller cingulate cortex volume and thicker temporal, instead, it was age-constant the volume enlargements in the frontal and parietal lobes. Another MRI study confirmed longitudinal progression of gray matter volume loss in NA-FEP but not in A-FEP [75].

Recently, Lewandowski et al. [76] suggested that major abnormalities in axon and myelin may not be pronounced in the very early phase of SCZ or BDP; instead, glial abnormalities are present, perhaps more intensely in patients with SCZ. These results have implications for the understanding of neuroprogressive processes in the early phases of diseases and into chronicity, and may be used to develop interventions targeting these processes while they are still sensitive to change. The authors focused on the role of glia in prefrontal white matter (WM) abnormalities in FEP or mania using a novel technique that allows the differentiation of myelin and axon measures using a combination of diffusion tensor spectroscopy (DTS) and magnetization transfer ratio (MRT). To our knowledge, this was the first study that applied combined MTR and DTS techniques in these populations to differentiate abnormalities of axon and myelin.

Equally interesting seems to be the investigation of connectivity strength (CS) analyzed by means of electroencephalogram (EEG) functional networks. CS estimates the degree of functional connectivity of the whole network and previous studies conducted on a sample of SCZ reported higher baseline CS values and modulation deficits in EEG spectral properties during cognitive activity [77, 78]. Cea-Cañas et al. [79] compared a sample of 171 subjects, SCZ and BPD patients and HC, focusing on theta and global frequency bands. They found a higher global band prestimulus CS in SCZ patients compared with BPD patients and HC and a highly significant deficit of theta band CS modulation in both SCZ and BPD. The larger global band pre-stimulus CS in SCZ was associated with worse cognitive performance, while lower theta band CS modulation was associated with negative symptoms [79]. Unfortunately, this study was conducted on a sample predominantly based on patients in chronic and stable phases of illness: only 31 were FEP patients. Further studies focusing on early stages of FEP could highlight if differences in CS may help understand future trajectories of these patients. This technique might represent a promising tool to anticipate a correct differential diagnosis at early stage of illness.

Auditory event-related potentials (ERPs) can be investigated using continuously recorded EEG. P3b is one of the most-studied ERPs in SCZ and it is well established that individuals with chronic SCZ show a robust reduction in its amplitude and can be considered both a trait and a state biomarker [80–82]. Patients with FEP and individuals at ultra-high risk for psychosis also show amplitude reductions [83–85]. Monaghan et al. [86] focused on a three-stimulus auditory oddball paradigm to elicit N1, P2, P3a, and P3b ERPs in a sample of 47 FEP patients (20 with SCZ spectrum diagnoses, 27 with BPD with psychotic features) and 29 HC subjects. They found that patients with BPD had a significantly larger baseline P2 amplitude than those with SCZ, corroborating previous findings from O'Donnell et al. [87] that showed reduced N1 and P2 amplitude in chronic SCZ but not BPD. These findings, if confirmed by future specific studies, suggest that P2 amplitude might distinguish between the two diagnostic categories.

Recently, Madeira et al. [88] conducted a study on a sample of 60 subjects, 20 patients with SCZ, 20 with BPD, in early years of disease, and 20 HC comparing groups with a combined approach of conventional and novel brain morphometric measures. They found an increased volume of the right globus pallidus in patients with SCZ, even at early stages of disease, and decreased gyrification of the right inferior frontal gyrus; divergent gyrification of the left supramarginal gyrus was found in patients with BPD vs. SCZ. These findings are in line with previous studies. Moreover, this brain MRI comparison study of individuals with SCZ or BPD in their first years of disease allowed to consider the increased volume of the right globus pallidus as a consistent marker in SCZ, but not BPD. On the other hand, compared with HC, they found increased gyrification of the left supramarginal gyrus (SMG) in patients with BPD and a decreased gyrification of the SMG in patients with SCZ. According to Kubota et al. [89], the reduced volume of SGM in SCZ could be negatively correlated with alexythimia in these patients and has been functionally associated to social cognition and Theory of Mind [90, 91]. Therefore, gyrification analysis, as an innovative and biologically plausible approach, could lead to identification of relevant biomarkers of different aspects of pathophysiology in SCZ and BPD. More studies using this approach in early-stage patients could enlighten specific disease trajectories, identifying distinct psychopathological phenotypes and its core neurobiological processes, maybe leading to helpful biomarkers for clinical practice, helping earlier diagnosis and improving treatment selection [88].

1.5 Prodromes

As we have seen, over the last decades, research on SCZ has tried to fulfill the need for early recognition and treatment of at-risk mental state. The effort to solve this necessity has been made also by recurring to retrospective studies. These studies have provided data about trajectories and symptoms in prodrome stage of illness, and according to 1–2 years follow-up data of multinational groups the rate of conversion from prodrome to full psychosis ranges between 15% and 40% [1].

Differently from studies on at-risk mental state for psychosis, research in BPD prodrome has concentrated largely on offspring of BPD patients, although the conversion rate among these subjects is low (3–10%) in follow-up studies [92]. Moreover, it should be considered that the majority of BPD patients do not have any parent with the same disorder. In order to identify adolescents and young adults at risk for developing BPD, it would be useful to recognize clinical symptoms that are indicative of transition, and to compare them with psychotic prodrome indicative of future SCZ diagnosis. Some findings point in this direction, nevertheless, more prospective studies on at-risk individuals are still needed in order to determine whether specific symptoms' clusters, either alone or in combination with endophenotypic markers, have sufficient predictive power to enable the clinical identification of patients at ultra-high risk for BPD.

According to current evidence, mania and SCZ prodrome's characteristics overlap considerably. Both can be described as a mixture of nonspecific psychopathology like a drop in social functioning, isolation, mood swings, and subthreshold symptoms of mania and/or depression [1]. Despite these similarities, a few differences can be highlighted.

Strange or unusual ideas, social isolation, and decreased school/work performance are the prevalent manifestations of SCZ prodrome [1, 93]. Attenuated positive symptoms have a key role in identifying future development of SCZ and mania with psychotic features; it appears that subthreshold hallucinations and delusions occur before in SCZ than in mania prodrome, while attenuated positive symptoms emerging late in the prodrome combined with increased energy/goal-directed activity are significantly more common in patients with later psychotic mania.

A relevant part of mania prodrome is represented by attenuated positive symptoms, particularly unusual thought content and difficulties in thinking/communicating clearly. Perceptual disturbances seem to be less frequent, when present attenuated auditory hallucinations are more common. These characteristics emerged from a retrospective study conducted by Correll et al. [1] based on 52 youths between 7 and 21 years old who had a diagnosis of BPD type I. Prodromal characteristics were compared between patients with and without subsequent psychotic mania and with known BPD and SCZ prodrome data. Schultze-Lutter et al. [93] found that the subthreshold negative symptoms-cluster is more represented in pre-SCZ patients: avolition, decreased ideational richness, decreased emotion expression and functioning deterioration obtained higher scores. Instead, physical agitation, depressive symptoms, suicidal thoughts, tiredness/lack of energy, decreased concentration/memory problems, difficulty thinking and obsessions/compulsions in mania prodrome are at least twice higher than in SCZ's. This group of patients showed an overall more severe psychopathology but not a more severe functional impairment [93]. Schultze-Lutter and colleagues reached these results with a naturalistic follow-up study, comparing prodromal symptoms of 74 patients who had sought help at an early detection center, and who, within 53 months on average, developed SCZ spectrum psychosis, affective disorder with psychotic features or affective disorder without psychotic features.

Burton et al. [94] conducted a longitudinal study in attenuated and early FEP, investigating the relationship between baseline psychopathology and longitudinal functional outcomes. According to their findings, worse negative symptoms or sub-threshold symptoms at baseline were strongly associated with worse social functioning across follow-up but this association decreased slightly over time, maybe as a result of treatment effects. Besides, the association between positive symptoms at baseline and social functioning reverses over time, being predictive of a long-term better social functioning outcome. Both associations supported the idea that negative and positive symptoms mutually affect social functioning, predicting a better outcome over time when present together. In fact, they highlighted the possibility that high symptoms on both dimensions might indicate the development of a disorder other than SCZ, but with a better prognosis, such as, for example, BPD. Particularly, thought disorder and negative symptoms appeared to be strongly related to functional outcomes up to 2 years follow-up in young people considered at high risk for psychosis, this relationship is very significant in order to address increasing attention to prevent not only conversion but also primarily functional impairment [94].

Interestingly, "grandiose ideas" play a controversial role: according to Schultze-Lutter et al. [93] exaggerated self-esteem is more frequent in future affective disorder than in future non-affective psychotic disorder, suggesting a key role of hypomanic symptoms in early detection of BPD. This finding contradicts previous results by Correll et al. [1] and Olvet et al. [43] that grandiose ideas appear to be more present in pre-psychotic disorder. It would be worthwhile to address more efforts to deepen this difference.

The discriminatory power of affective dimensions (manic, activation, dysphoric, and depressive) have been investigated by Arrasate et al. [95]. According to their findings, the activation dimension alone, or combined with the manic one, showed the best predictive value for BPD diagnosis in FEP patients to the point that if they had been used together the 64% of BPD patients who got a delayed diagnosis could have correctly detected from the beginning. Furthermore, the dysphoric dimension seems to be a relevant factor in discrimination between BPD and other psychoses. These results came from a prospective, longitudinal study conducted over 112 patients with FEP, followed-up for 5 years.

These symptom clusters have been also investigated in children's psychiatry departments; "abnormal suspiciousness or sensitivity" and "extrafamilial relationship difficulties" seem to be strongly associated with later SCZ. Instead, the "hysterical symptom-cluster" (such as depersonalization, conversive symptoms, and non-epileptic disturbance of consciousness) "hypochondriasis," "disturbance of eating," and "gross overactivity" are associated to future affective psychosis. For both, SCZ and affective psychosis, speech and language disturbance have no predictive value [96].

Even if some of the current findings seem to be promising, at the current state of the art many of the abovementioned symptom clusters are very nonspecific to become solid predictors of development of later SCZ or BPD. Clearly, more prospective studies on at-risk subjects are necessary.

More recently few studies have examined the occurrence of psychotic symptoms in adolescent-onset BPD. Child and adolescent psychiatry clinicians tended to overlook affective manifestations in patients with psychotic symptoms or to poorly investigate disorganization and psychotic symptoms in mood disorders, generating diagnostic uncertainty between BPD and SCZ [97, 98].

Fu-I et al. [99] investigated the frequency of psychotic and affective symptoms during the first manic episode, their findings suggest that disorganization and psychotic symptoms during the first manic episode are key features in adolescent onset of BPD, and that psychotic depression frequently may precede psychotic mania. The study was conducted on a sample of 49 adolescents with BPD type I admitted to the hospital during their first acute manic episode. As it would be expected, these patients exhibited typical manic features such as psychomotor agitation, grandiosity, and euphoria. In addition, disorganization and psychotic symptoms were present in 55% of the total sample. Interestingly, most patients (76%) reported at least one previous depressive episode; of these, 47% had prominent psychotic features [99]. Nevertheless, the reliability of differential diagnosis between BPD and SCZ in children and adolescents remain a source of debate. This confusion often delays treatment for both disorders, that is why further investigations focused on disorganization symptoms during depressive episodes in children and adolescents are needed to help differentiate unipolar depressive episode, BDP, and SCZ [99–101].

1.6 Conclusions

The discussion presented in this chapter focused on the importance of early identifying the evolution of FEP, toward SCZ and BPD. Even though researchers are currently seeking to respond to this unmet need, it is possible to highlight some tools which might help clinicians to better understand the possible trajectories of patients with FEP. GWA studies seem to be promising in estimating PRS that can be used to predict outcomes of these patients. Quality and quantity of cognitive impairment might suggest trajectories of FEP patients and high-risk individuals; in fact, it appears that lower QI scores in premorbid and first phase of illness are typical of SCZ, rather than BPD. Specific neurocognitive domains might be involved in differential diagnosis, such as verbal fluency; whether confirmed by further investigations, it could become a strong diagnostic marker for SCZ. Neuroimaging investigations in the field of mental disorders represent a very promising aspect of psychiatric research; not only fMRI, but also EEG could provide useful information to allow early differentiation of FEP's trajectories. Finally, an important breakthrough would be to identify specific clinical features of prodrome states suggestive of future affective or non-affective diagnosis. A few differences can be highlighted: subthreshold negative symptoms appear to be more represented in SCZ, whereas physical agitation, concentration and memory problems, suicidal thoughts, difficulty thinking, and obsessions/compulsions in mania prodrome are at least twice high than in SCZs. Grandiose ideas and dysphoric dimension seem to suggest a future BPD diagnosis. The reliability of differential diagnosis in children and adolescents is still a source of debate, to solve this issue would be the key to allow early diagnosis and to avoid treatment delays.

References

1. Correll CU, Penzner JB, Frederickson AM, Richter JJ, Author AM, Smith CW, Kane JM, Cornblatt BA. Differentiation in the preonset phases of schizophrenia and mood disorders: evidence in support of a bipolar mania prodrome. Schizophr Bull. 2007;33:703–14.
2. Geoffroy PA, Leboyer M, Scott J. [Predicting bipolar disorder: what can we learn from prospective cohort studies?]. Encephale. 2015;41(1):10–6.
3. Hammerschlag AR, de Leeuw CA, Middeldorp CM, Polderman TJC. Synaptic and brain-expressed gene sets relate to the shared genetic risk across five psychiatric disorders. Psychol Med. 2020;50(10):1695–705.
4. Torrent C, Reinares M, Martinez-Aran A, Cabrera B, Amoretti S, Corripio I, et al. Affective versus non-affective first episode psychoses: a longitudinal study. J Affect Disord. 2018;238:297–304.
5. Correll CU, Galling B, Pawar A, Krivko A, Bonetto C, Ruggeri M, et al. Comparison of early intervention services vs treatment as usual for early-phase psychosis: a systematic review, meta-analysis, and meta-regression effectiveness of early intervention services for early-phase psychosis effectiveness of early intervention services for early-phase psychosis. JAMA Psychiat. 2018;75(6):555–65.
6. Kane JM, Robinson DG, Schooler NR, Mueser KT, Penn DL, Rosenheck RA, Addington J, Brunette MF, Correll CU, Estroff SE, Marcy P, Robinson J, Meyer-Kalos PS, Gottlieb JD, Glynn SM, Lynde DW, Pipes R, Kurian BT, Miller AL, Azrin ST, Goldstein AB, Severe JB, Lin H, Sint KJ, John M, Heinssen RK. Comprehensive versus usual community care for first-episode psychosis: 2-year outcomes from the NIMH RAISE early treatment program. Am J Psychiatry. 2016;173(4):362–72.
7. Kane JM, Schooler NR, Marcy P, Correll CU, Brunette MF, Mueser KT, Rosenheck RA, Addington J, Estroff SE, Robinson J, Penn DL, Robinson DG. The RAISE early treatment program for first-episode psychosis: background, rationale, and study design. J Clin Psychiatry. 2015;76(3):240–6.
8. Mueser KT, Penn DL, Addington J, Brunette MF, Gingerich S, Glynn SM, Lynde DW, Gottlieb JD, Meyer-Kalos P, McGurk SR, Cather C, Saade S, Robinson DG, Schooler NR, Rosenheck RA, Kane JM. The NAVIGATE program for first episode psychosis: rationale, overview, and description of psychosocial components. Psychiatr Serv. 2015;66(7):680–90.
9. Addington J, Chaves A, Addington D. Diagnostic stability over one year in first-episode psychosis. Schizophr Res. 2006;86(1–3):71–5.
10. Fusar-Poli P, Cappucciati M, Rutigliano G, Heslin M, Stahl D, Brittenden Z, Caverzasi E, McGuire P, Carpenter WT. Diagnostic stability of ICD/-DSM first episode psychosis diagnoses: meta-analysis. Schizophr Bull. 2016;42(6):1395–406.

11. Cawkwell PB, Bolton KW, Karmacharya R, Öngür D, Shinn AK. Two-year diagnostic stability in a real-world sample of individuals with early psychosis. Early Interv Psychiatry. 2020;14(6):751–4.
12. Goldstein BI, Birmaher B, Carlson GA, DelBello MP, Findling RL, Fristad M, et al. The International Society for Bipolar Disorders Task Force report on pediatric bipolar disorder: knowledge to date and directions for future research. Bipolar Disord. 2017;19:524–43.
13. Morgan C, Lappin J, Heslin M, Donoghue K, Lomas B, Reininghaus U, Onyejiaka A, Jones PB, Murray RM, Fearon P, Doody GA, Dazzan P. Reappraising the long-term course and outcome of psychotic disorders: the AESOP-10 study. Psychol Med. 2014;44(13):2713–26.
14. Suvisaari J, Mantere O, Keinanen J, Mantyla T, Rikandi E, Lindgren M, et al. Is it possible to predict the future in first-episode psychosis? Front Psych. 2018;9:580.
15. Green EK, Raybould R, Macgregor S, Gordon-Smith K, Heron J, Hyde S, Grozeva D, Hamshere M, Williams N, Owen MJ, O'Donovan MC, Jones L, Jones I, Kirov G, Craddock N. Operation of the schizophrenia susceptibility gene, neuregulin 1, across traditional diagnostic boundaries to increase risk for bipolar disorder. Arch Gen Psychiatry. 2005;62:642–52.
16. Moskvina V, Craddock N, Holmas P, Nikolov I. Gene-wide analyses of genome-wide association data sets: evidence for multiple common risk alleles for schizophrenia and bipolar disorder and overlap in genetic risk. Mol Psychiatry. 2009;14:252–60.
17. Shao L, Vawter MP. Shared gene expression alterations in schizophrenia and bipolar disorder. Biol Psychiatry. 2008;64:89–97.
18. Craddock N, O'Donovan MC, Owen MJ. Psychosis genetics: modeling the relationship between schizophrenia, bipolar disorder, and mixed (or "schizoaffective") psychoses. Schizophr Bull. 2009;35:482–90.
19. Carroll LS, Owen MJ. Genetic overlap between autism, schizophrenia and bipolar disorder. Genome Med. 2009;1:1–102.
20. Grozeva D, Kirov G, Ivanov D, Jones IR. Rare copy number variants: a point of rarity in genetic risk for bipolar disorder and schizophrenia. Arch Gen Psychiatry. 2010;67:318–27.
21. Emamian ES, Hall D, Birnbaum MJ, Karayiorgou M, Gogos JA. Convergent evidence for impaired AKT1-GSK3beta signaling in schizophrenia. Nat Genet. 2004;36:131–7.
22. Thiselton DL, Vladimirov VI, Kuo PH, McClay J, Wormley B, Fanous A, O'Neill FA, Walsh D, Van den Oord EJ, Kendler KS, Riley BP. AKT1 is associated with schizophrenia across multiple symptom dimensions in the Irish study of high density schizophrenia families. Biol Psychiatry. 2008;63:449–57.
23. Toyota T, Yamada K, Detera-Wadleigh SD, Yoshikawa T. Analysis of a cluster of polymorphisms in AKT1 gene in bipolar pedigrees: a family-based association study. Neurosci Lett. 2003;339:5–8.
24. Karege F, Méary A, Perroud N, Jamain S, Leboyer M, Ballmann E, Schürhoff F. Genetic overlap between schizophrenia and bipolar disorder: a study with AKT1 gene variants and clinical phenotypes. Schizophr Res. 2012;135(1–3):8–14.
25. Farrell MS, Werge T, Sklar P, Owen MJ, Ophoff RA, O'Donovan MC, Corvin A, Cichon S, Sullivan PF. Evaluating historical candidate genes for schizophrenia. Mol Psychiatry. 2015;20:555–62.
26. Johnson EC, Border R, Melroy-Greif WE, de Leeuw CA, Ehringer MA, Keller MC. No evidence that schizophrenia candidate genes are more associated with schizophrenia than non-candidate genes. Biol Psychiatry. 2017;82:702–8.
27. Wray NR, Goddard ME, Visscher PM. Prediction of individual genetic risk to disease from genome-wide association studies. Genome Res. 2007;17(10):1520–8.
28. Purcell SM, Wray NR, Stone JL, Visscher PM, O'Donovan MC, et al. Common polygenic variation contributes to risk of schizophrenia and bipolar disorder. Nature. 2009;460:748–52.
29. Ripke S, Sanders AR, Kendler KS, Levinson DF, Sklar P, et al. Genome-wide association study identifies five new schizophrenia loci. Nat Genet. 2011;43:969–76.
30. Dudbridge F. Power and predictive accuracy of polygenic risk scores. PLoS Genet. 2013;9(3):e1003348.

31. Allardyce J, Leonenko G, Hamshere M, Pardiñas AF, Forty L, Knott S, et al. Association between schizophrenia-related polygenic liability and the occurrence and level of mood-incongruent psychotic symptoms in bipolar disorder. JAMA Psychiat. 2018;75:28–35.
32. Bipolar Disorder and Schizophrenia Working Group of the Psychiatric Genomics Consortium. Genomic dissection of bipolar disorder and schizophrenia, including 28 subphenotypes. Cell. 2018;173:1705–15.
33. Millan MJ, Agid Y, Brune M, Bullmore ET, Carter CS, Clayton NS, Connor R, Davis S, Deakin B, DeRubeis RJ, Dubois B, Geyer MA, Goodwin GM, Gorwood P, Jay TM, Joels M, Mansuy IM, Meyer-Lindenberg A, et al. Cognitive dysfunction in psychiatric disorders: characteristics, causes and the quest for improved therapy. Nat Rev Drug Discov. 2012;11(2):141–68.
34. Depp CA, Mausbach BT, Harmell AL, Savla GN, Bowie CR, Harvey PD, Patterson TL. Meta-analysis of the association between cognitive abilities and everyday functioning in bipolar disorder. Bipolar Disord. 2012;14(3):217–26.
35. Green MF, Horan WP, Lee J. Nonsocial and social cognition in schizophrenia: current evidence and future directions. World Psychiatry. 2019;18(2):146–61.
36. Sheffield JM, Karcher NR, Barch DM. Cognitive deficits in psychotic disorders: a lifespan perspective. Neuropsychol Rev. 2018;28(4):509–33.
37. Stefanopoulou E, Manoharan A, Landau S, Geddes JR, Goodwin G, Frangou S. Cognitive functioning in patients with affective disorders and schizophrenia: a meta-analysis. Int Rev Psychiatry. 2009;21(4):336–56.
38. Yen CF, Cheng CP, Huang CF, Ko CH, Yen JY, Chang YP, Chen CS. Relationship between psychosocial adjustment and executive function in patients with bipolar disorder and schizophrenia in remission: the mediating and moderating effects of insight. Bipolar Disord. 2009;11(2):190–7.
39. Cuesta MJ, Sanchez-Torres AM, Cabrera B, Bioque M, Merchan-Naranjo J, Corripio I, Gonzalez-Pinto A, Lobo A, Bombin I, de la Serna E, Sanjuan J, Parellada M, Saiz-Ruiz J, Bernardo M. Premorbid adjustment and clinical correlates of cognitive impairment in first-episode psychosis. The PEPsCog Study. Schizophr Res. 2015a;164(1–3):65–73.
40. Lewandowski KE, Cohen BM, Keshavan MS, Ongur D. Relationship of neurocognitive deficits to diagnosis and symptoms across affective and non-affective psychoses. Schizophr Res. 2011a;133(1–3):212–7.
41. Lewandowski KE, Cohen BM, Ongur D. Evolution of neuropsychological dysfunction during the course of schizophrenia and bipolar disorder. Psychol Med. 2011b;41(2):225–41.
42. Trotta A, Murray RM, MacCabe JH. Do premorbid and post-onset cognitive functioning differ between schizophrenia and bipolar disorder? A systematic review and meta-analysis. Psychol Med. 2015;45(2):381–94.
43. Olvet DM, Stearns WH, McLaughlin D, Auther AM, Correll CU, Cornblatt BA. Comparing clinical and neurocognitive features of the schizophrenia prodrome to the bipolar prodrome. Schizophr Res. 2010;123(1):59–63.
44. Seidman LJ, Giuliano AJ, Smith CW, Stone WS, Glatt SJ, Meyer E, Faraone SV, Tsuang MT, Cornblatt B. Neuropsychological functioning in adolescents and young adults at genetic risk for schizophrenia and affective psychoses: results from the Harvard and Hillside Adolescent High Risk Studies. Schizophr Bull. 2006;32(3):507–24.
45. Maziade M, Rouleau N, Gingras N, et al. Shared neurocognitive dysfunctions in young offspring at extreme risk for schizophrenia or bipolar disorder in eastern Quebec multigenerational families. Schizophr Bull. 2009;35:919–30.
46. Woodberry KA, Giuliano AJ, Seidman LJ. Premorbid IQ in schizophrenia: a meta-analytic review. Am J Psychiatry. 2008;165(5):579–87.
47. Martino DJ, Samame C, Ibanez A, Strejilevich SA. Neurocognitive functioning in the premorbid stage and in the first episode of bipolar disorder: a systematic review. Psychiatry Res. 2015;226(1):23–30.
48. Mollon J, Reichenberg A. Cognitive development prior to onset of psychosis. Psychol Med. 2017;48(3):392–403.

49. Parellada M, Gomez-Vallejo S, Burdeus M, Arango C. Developmental differences between schizophrenia and bipolar disorder. Schizophr Bull. 2017;43(6):1176–89.
50. Cannon M, Caspi A, Moffitt TE, Harrington H, Taylor A, Murray RM, et al. Evidence for early-childhood, pan-developmental impairment specific to schizophreniform disorder: results from a longitudinal birth cohort. Arch Gen Psychiatry. 2002;59(5):449–56.
51. Sorensen HJ, Saebye D, Urfer-Parnas A, Mortensen EL, Parnas J. Premorbid intelligence and educational level in bipolar and unipolar disorders: a Danish draft board study. J Affect Disord. 2012;136(3):1188–91.
52. Zammit S, Allebeck P, David AS, Dalman C, Hemmingsson T, Lundberg I, et al. A longitudinal study of premorbid IQ Score and risk of developing schizophrenia, bipolar disorder, severe depression, and other nonaffective psychoses. Arch Gen Psychiatry. 2004;61(4):354–60.
53. Grande I, Berk M, Birmaher B, Vieta E. Bipolar disorder. Lancet. 2016;387(10027):1561–72.
54. Kumar CT, Frangou S. Clinical implications of cognitive function in bipolar disorder. Ther Adv Chronic Dis. 2010;1(3):85–93.
55. MacCabe JH, Wicks S, Lofving S, David AS, Berndtsson A, Gustafsson JE, et al. Decline in cognitive performance between ages 13 and 18 years and the risk for psychosis in adulthood: a Swedish longitudinal cohort study in males. JAMA Psychiatry. 2013;70(3):261–70.
56. Tiihonen J, Haukka J, Henriksson M, Cannon M, Kieseppa T, Laaksonen I, et al. Premorbid intellectual functioning in bipolar disorder and schizophrenia: results from a cohort study of male conscripts. Am J Psychiatry. 2005;162(10):1904–10.
57. Koenen KC, Moffitt TE, Roberts AL, Martin LT, Kubzansky L, Harrington H, Poulton R, Caspi A. Childhood IQ and adult mental disorders: a test of the cognitive reserve hypothesis. Am J Psychiatry. 2009;166(1):50–7.
58. Daban C, Martinez-Aran A, Torrent C, Tabares-Seisdedos R, Balanza-Martinez V, Salazar-Fraile J, et al. Specificity of cognitive deficits in bipolar disorder versus schizophrenia. A systematic review. Psychother Psychosom. 2006;75(2):72–84.
59. Paya B, Rodriguez-Sanchez JM, Otero S, Munoz P, Castro-Fornieles J, Parellada M, et al. Premorbid impairments in early-onset psychosis: differences between patients with schizophrenia and bipolar disorder. Schizophr Res. 2013;146(1–3):103–10.
60. Kendler KS, Ohlsson H, Mezuk B, Sundquist K, Sundquist J. A Swedish National Prospective and co-relative study of school achievement at age 16, and risk for schizophrenia, other non-affective psychosis, and bipolar illness. Schizophr Bull. 2016;42(1):77–86.
61. Seidman LJ, Cherkerzian S, Goldstein JM, Agnew-Blais J, Tsuang MT, Buka SL. Neuropsychological performance and family history in children at age 7 who develop adult schizophrenia or bipolar psychosis in the New England Family Studies. Psychol Med. 2013;43(1):119–31.
62. Amoretti S, Bernardo M, Bonnin CM, Bioque M, Cabrera B, Mezquida G, Sole B, Vieta E, Torrent C. The impact of cognitive reserve in the outcome of first-episode psychoses: 2-year follow-up study. Eur Neuropsychopharmacol. 2016;26(10):1638–48.
63. Anaya C, Torrent C, Caballero FF, Vieta E, Bonnin CM, Ayuso-Mateos JL. Cognitive reserve in bipolar disorder: relation to cognition, psychosocial functioning and quality of life. Acta Psychiatr Scand. 2016;133(5):386–98.
64. Grande I, Sanchez-Moreno J, Sole B, Jimenez E, Torrent C, Bonnin CM, Varo C, Tabares-Seisdedos R, Balanza-Martinez V, Valls E, Morilla I, Carvalho AF, Ayuso-Mateos JL, Vieta E, Martinez-Aran A. High cognitive reserve in bipolar disorders as a moderator of neurocognitive impairment. J Affect Disord. 2017;208:621–7.
65. Gonzalez-Ortega I, de los Mozos V, Echeburua E, Mezo M, Besga A, Ruiz de Azua S, Gonzalez-Pinto A, Gutierrez M, Zorrilla I, Gonzalez-Pinto A. Working memory as a predictor of negative symptoms and functional outcome in first episode psychosis. Psychiatry Res. 2013;206(1):8–16.
66. Harvey PD, Green MF, Bowie C, Loebel A. The dimensions of clinical and cognitive change in schizophrenia: evidence for independence of improvements. Psychopharmacology. 2006;187(3):356–63.

67. Costafreda SG, Fu CH, Picchioni M, Toulopoulou T, McDonald C, Kravariti E, Walshe M, Prata D, Murray RM, McGuire PK. Pattern of neural responses to verbal fluency shows diagnostic specificity for schizophrenia and bipolar disorder. BMC Psychiatry. 2011;11(18):18–1.
68. Raucher-Chene D, Achim AM, Kaladjian A, Besche-Richard C. Verbal fluency in bipolar disorders: a systematic review and meta-analysis. J Affect Disord. 2017;207:359–66.
69. Berger GE, Bartholomeusz CF, Wood SJ, Ang A, Phillips LJ, Proffitt T, Brewer WJ, Smith DJ, Nelson B, Lin A, Borgwardt S, Velakoulis D, Yung AR, McGorry PD, Pantelis C. Ventricular volumes across stages of schizophrenia and other psychoses. Aust N Z J Psychiatry. 2017;51:1041–51.
70. Chung Y, Haut KM, He G, Van Erp TG, McEwen S, Addington J, Bearden CE, Cadenhead K, Cornblatt B, Mathalon DH, McGlashan T, Perkins D, Seidman LJ, Tsuang M, Walker E. Ventricular enlargement and progressive reduction of cortical gray matter are linked in prodromal youth who develop psychosis. Schizophr Res. 2017;189:169–74.
71. Vita A, De Peri L, Sacchetti E. Gray matter, white matter, brain, and intracranial volumes in first-episode bipolar disorder: a meta-analysis of magnetic resonance imaging studies. Bipolar Disord. 2009;11:807–14.
72. Calvo A, Delvecchio G, Altamura AC, Soares JC, Brambilla P. Gray matter volume differences between affective and non-affective first episode psychosis: a review of magnetic resonance imaging studies. J Affect Disord. 2018;243:564–74.
73. Vita A, De Peri L, Silenzi C, Dieci M. Brain morphology in first-episode schizophrenia: a meta-analysis of quantitative magnetic resonance imaging studies. Schizophr Res. 2006;82:75–88.
74. Pina-Camacho L, Del Rey-Mejìas Á, Janssen J, Bioque M, Gonzulez-Pinto A, Arango C, Lobo A, Sarrò S, Desco M, Sanjuan J, Cuesta M, Saiz-Ruiz J, Bernardo M, Paradella M, Lacalle-Aurioles M. Age at first episode modulates diagnosis-related structural brain abnormalities in psychosis. Schizophr Bull. 2016;42(2):344–57.
75. Ohtani T, Del Re E, Levitt JJ, Niznikiewicz M, Konishi J, Asami T, Kawashima T, Roppongi T, Nestor PG, Shenton ME, McCarley RW, Salisbury DF. Progressive symptom-associated prefrontal volume loss occurs in first-episode schizophrenia but not in affective psychosis. Brain Struct Funct. 2018;223(6):2879–92.
76. Lewandowski KE, Du F, Fan X, Chen X, Huynh P, Öngur D. Role of glia in prefrontal white matter abnormalities in first episode psychosis or mania detected by diffusion tensor spectroscopy. Schizophr Res. 2019;209:64–71.
77. Gomez-Pilar J, Lubeiro A, Poza J, Hornero R, Ayuso M, Valcarcel C, Haidar K, Blanco JA, Molina V. Functional EEG network analysis in schizophrenia: evidence of larger segregation and deficit of modulation. Prog Neuropsychopharmacol Biol Psychiatry. 2017;76:116–23.
78. Gomez-Pilar J, de Luis-Garcia R, Lubeiro A, de la Red H, Poza J, Nuñez P, Hornero R, Molina V. Relations between structural and EEG-based graph metrics in healthy controls and schizophrenia patients. Hum Brain Mapp. 2018;39(8):3152–65.
79. Cea-Cañas B, Gomez-Pilar J, Nuñez P, Rodriguez-Vazquez E, de Uribe N, Diez Á, et al. Connectivity strength of the EEG functional network in schizophrenia and bipolar disorder. Prog Neuro-Psychopharmacol Biol Psychiatry. 2020;98:109801.
80. Bramon E, Rabe-Hesketh S, Sham P, Murray RM, Frangou S. Meta-analysis of the P300 and P50 waveforms in schizophrenia. Schizophr Res. 2004;70:315–29.
81. Jeon YW, Polich J. P300 asymmetry in schizophrenia: a meta-analysis. Psychiatry Res. 2001;104:61–74.
82. Polich J, Jeon YW. Meta-analysis of P300 and schizophrenia: patients, paradigms, and practical implications. Psychophysiology. 2003;40:684–701.
83. del Re EC, Spencer KM, Oribe N, Mesholam-Gately RI, Goldstein J, Shenton ME, Petryshen T, Seidman LJ, McCarley RW, Niznikiewicz MA. Clinical high risk and first episode schizophrenia: auditory event-related potentials. Psychiatry Res. 2015;231:126–33.
84. Morales-Muñoz I, Jurado-Barba R, Fernández-Guinea S, Álvarez-Alonso MJ, Rodríguez-Jiménez R, Jiménez-Arriero MA, Rubio G. Cognitive impairments in patients with first

episode psychosis: the relationship between neurophysiological and neuropsychological assessments. J Clin Neurosci. 2017;36:80–7.
85. van Tricht MJ, Nieman DH, Koelman JHTM, Bour LJ, van der Meer JN, van Amelsvoort TA, Linszen DH, de Haan L. Auditory ERP components before and after transition to a first psychotic episode. Biol Psychol. 2011;87:350–7.
86. Monaghan CK, Brickman S, Huynh P, Öngur D, Hall MH. A longitudinal study of event related potentials and correlations with psychosocial functioning and clinical features in first episode psychosis patients. Int J Psychophysiol. 2019;145:48–56.
87. O'Donnell BF, Vohs JL, Hetrick WP, Carroll CA, Shekhar A. Auditory event-related potential abnormalities in bipolar disorder and schizophrenia. Int J Psychophysiol. 2004;53:45–55.
88. Madeira N, Duarte JV, Martins R, Costa GN, Macedo A, Castelo-Branco M. Morphometry and gyrification in bipolar disorder and schizophrenia: a comparative MRI study. NeuroImage Clin. 2020;26:102220.
89. Kubota M, Miyata J, Yoshida H, Hirao K, Fujiwara H, Kawada R, Fujimoto S, Tanaka Y, Sasamoto A, Sawamoto N, Fukuyama H, Murai T. Age-related cortical thinning in schizophrenia. Schizophr Res. 2011;125:21–9.
90. Saxe R, Powell LJ. It's the thought that counts: specific brain regions for one component of theory of mind. Psychol Sci. 2006;17:692–9.
91. Silani G, Lamm C, Ruff CC, Singer T. Right supramarginal gyrus is crucial to overcome emotional egocentricity bias in social judgments. J Neurosci. 2013;33:15466–76.
92. Hillegers MH, Reichart CG, Wals M, Verhulst FC, Ormel J, Nolen WA. Five-year prospective outcome of psychopathology in the adolescent offspring of bipolar parents. Bipolar Disord. 2005;7(4):344–50.
93. Schultze-Lutter F, Schimmelmann BG, Klosterkötter J, Ruhrmann S. Comparing the prodrome of schizophrenia-spectrum psychoses and affective disorders with and without psychotic features. Schizophr Res. 2012;138(2–3):218–22.
94. Burton CZ, Tso IF, Carrión RE, Niendam T, Adelsheim S, Auther AM, Cornblatt BA, Carter CS, Melton R, Sale TG, Taylor SF, McFarlane WR. Baseline psychopathology and relationship to longitudinal functional outcome in attenuated and early first episode psychosis. Schizophr Res. 2019;212:157–62.
95. Arrasate M, Gonzalez-Ortega I, Alberich S, Gutierrez M, Martinez-Cengotitabengoa M, Mosquera F, Cruz N, Gonzalez-Torres MA, Henry C, González-Pinto A. Affective dimensions as a diagnostic tool for bipolar disorder in first psychotic episodes. Eur Psychiatry. 2014;29:424–30.
96. Cannon M, Walsh E, Hollis C, Kargin M, Taylor E, Murray RM, Jones PB. Predictors of later schizophrenia and affective psychosis among attendees at a child psychiatry department. Br J Psychiatry. 2001;178(5):420–6.
97. Correll CU, Hauser M, Penzner JB, Auther AM, Kafantaris V, Saito E, et al. Type and duration of subsyndromal symptoms in youth with bipolar I disorder prior to their first manic episode. Bipolar Disord. 2014;16:478–92.
98. Parellada M, Castro-Fornieles J, Gonzalez-Pinto A, Pina-Camacho L, Moreno D, Rapado-Castro M, et al. Predictors of functional and clinical outcome in early-onset first-episode psychosis: the child and adolescent first episode of psychosis (CAFEPS) study. J Clin Psychiatry. 2015;76:e1441–8.
99. Fu-I L, Gurgel WDS, Caetano SC, Machado-Vieira R, Wang YP. Psychotic and affective symptoms of early-onset bipolar disorder: an observational study of patients in first manic episode. Braz J Psychiatry. 2019;42(2):168–74.
100. Leopold K, Ratzer S, Correll CU, Rottmann-Wolf M, Pfeiffer S, Ritter P, et al. Characteristics, symptomatology and naturalistic treatment in individuals at-risk for bipolar disorders: baseline results in the first 180 help-seeking individuals assessed at the Dresden high-risk project. J Affect Disord. 2014;152–154:427–33.
101. Reimherr JP, McClellan JM. Diagnostic challenges in children and adolescents with psychotic disorders. J Clin Psychiatry. 2004;65:5–11.

2 New Strategies to Improve Cognitive Symptom Domain in the Treatment of Schizophrenia

Stefano Barlati, Cassandra Ariu, Andrea Garozzo, and Antonio Vita

2.1 Introduction

Cognitive impairment, in past decades, has been consistently reported in patients with schizophrenia [1]. Neurocognitive disability appears early in the course of the disease, even in prodromal phases, and these deficits are widely present in different stages of the illness whether in patients or in their first-degree family members [2]. In 2004, the Measurement and Treatment Research to Improve Cognition in Schizophrenia (MATRICS) project has identified seven distinct cognitive domains that are impaired in patients with schizophrenia: speed of processing, attention/vigilance, working memory, verbal and visual learning, reasoning and problem solving, and social cognition [3–5]. Moreover, in the third meeting of the Cognitive Neuroscience Treatment Research to Improve Cognition in Schizophrenia (CNTRICS) project, it was cleared that six areas of cognitive domains are damaged in patients with schizophrenia: perception, working memory, attention, executive functions, long-term memory, and social cognition [6]. Regarding social cognitive deficits, they include impairments in facial affect recognition, in perceiving and interpreting social cues, in theory of mind (ToM), and in the ability to make appropriate causal attributions for events [7]. Several studies have shown that both neurocognitive and social cognitive deficits are among the major causes of severe

S. Barlati · A. Vita (✉)
Department of Mental Health and Addiction Services, ASST Spedali Civili of Brescia, Brescia, Italy

Department of Clinical and Experimental Sciences, University of Brescia, Brescia, Italy
e-mail: antonio.vita@unibs.it

C. Ariu
Department of Mental Health and Addiction Services, ASST Spedali Civili of Brescia, Brescia, Italy

A. Garozzo
Department of Mental Health and Addiction Services, ASST of Mantova, Mantova, Italy

P. Rocca, S. Bellino (eds.), *Psychosis and Personality Disorders*,
https://doi.org/10.1007/978-3-031-09058-5_2

functional disabilities in patients with schizophrenia and they are also related to a worse outcome of the disorder [8–10]. In a comprehensive literature review, Green et al. [10] underlined that different cognitive deficits might have an impact on specific areas of psychosocial functioning. As a matter of fact, cognitive deficits seem to explain 20–60% of the variance of everyday functioning [3, 4, 11]. The influence of cognition on functional outcomes may happen through its influence on functional capacity, the ability to perform critical everyday living skills [12]. Thus, functional capacity may actually be considered as a proxy measure between neurocognition and everyday functioning and it has been found to be quite strongly associated with cognitive performance [13]. Recent studies have shown how cognitive impairment predicts functional outcomes even more than positive and negative symptoms and how it is associated with disability in phases of clinical remission too [2, 14]. From the greater and detailed knowledge of the role and meaning of cognitive impairment in schizophrenia, its improvement became an essential target in the treatment and in the clinical management of the illness [15]. In order to restore cognitive deficits in schizophrenic patients, there are different pharmacological and non-pharmacological approaches developed. Whereas pharmacological interventions include approved treatments (e.g., antipsychotics and antidepressants) and under-study treatments, non-pharmacological interventions include cognitive remediation, noninvasive brain stimulation techniques, and physical activity techniques [16–20].

This chapter will focus on the analysis of various pharmacological treatments and of cognitive remediation techniques, as regards to non-pharmacological interventions. We decided to not include in the chapter other non-pharmacological (e.g., aerobic physical exercise) and/or somatic (e.g., brain stimulation) techniques potentially effective, or at least promising, for improving cognitive functioning in schizophrenia. Our aim is to increase the knowledge and understanding of the principles and methodology of these interventions for schizophrenia and to highlight the evidence of effectiveness of such interventions deriving from the current scientific literature.

2.2 Pharmacological Treatment to Improve Cognitive Functioning in Schizophrenia

2.2.1 Cognitive Functioning in Schizophrenia: Focus on Treatment Management

An important prerequisite for the success of cognitive enhancement interventions in schizophrenia is the stabilization of symptoms through optimal use of antipsychotics and other psychotropic medications [21]. An ideal pharmacotherapy includes a global assessment, an integrated care plan, and careful attention to therapeutic alliance, in addition to an appropriate choice of the medication(s), adherence, evaluation of comorbidities, and side effects. Avoiding unnecessary or excessive use of medications, as well as reducing the use of drugs with possible negative cognitive effects (for example, anticholinergics), could lead to cognitive benefits [21].

2.2.2 Cognitive Functioning in Schizophrenia: Focus on Metabolic Profile

The relationship between cognition and the metabolic side effects of antipsychotic medications is complicated. The available literature regarding this topic is sparse, but it suggests a relationship between metabolic comorbidities and worse cognitive function in patients with schizophrenia [22]. Generally, the impact of the metabolic syndrome on cognitive functions is more pronounced in patients with severe negative symptoms [23–26]. Meta-analyses have further confirmed the effects of metabolic syndrome and type II diabetes mellitus (T2DM) as determinants of poor overall cognition in schizophrenia [27]. Better cognitive performance at baseline has also been associated with a favorable metabolic profile at follow-up in schizophrenia [28]. Individual metabolic syndrome constituent components may exert distinct effects on specific cognitive domains in schizophrenia. For example, a higher waist circumference has been correlated with decreased motor speed [24] and attention/vigilance [26], while hypertension and elevated triglycerides have been associated with poorer verbal memory [29, 30]. This relationship appears to be very important, considering the increased risk of developing metabolic syndrome in schizophrenic patients [31].

2.2.3 Cognitive Functioning in Schizophrenia: Focus on First- and Second-Generation Antipsychotics

Treatment with antipsychotics in schizophrenia is often limited to the reduction of positive symptoms, while negative symptoms and cognitive impairment may persist throughout life [32]. First-generation antipsychotics (FGAs), especially, have relatively little influence on cognitive and negative symptoms and may cause adverse side effects, such as extrapyramidal motor symptoms (EPS), tardive dyskinesia, weight gain, and sedation [33]. More specifically, FGAs treatment seems to improve certain executive functions in the short period, but there is a decline relative to baseline of moderate-to-large effect size (ES) in the long period [34] and, finally, long-term treatment with FGAs can cause cognitive deterioration as a side effect [35]. More specifically, in the randomized NeSSy trial, second-generation antipsychotics (SGAs) presented an advantage over FGAs in cognitive function during medium-term treatment for schizophrenia. Findings also highlighted a distinction between progression to the harmful effects of FGAs with prolonged treatment as opposed to more persistent cognitive benefits with SGAs treatment [34]. This is in line with recent findings from meta-analysis studies on neuroimaging and antipsychotics in schizophrenia patients [36]. SGAs drugs may partially improve cognitive dysfunction, which may be related to their relatively high affinity for serotonin 5HT2A receptors compared with D2 receptors [37]. The apparent cognitive enhancement may be related to one or more of the following effects of atypical antipsychotics agents, not shared by FGAs: increased release of dopamine (DA) and acetylcholine (ACh) in the prefrontal cortex (PFC) and hippocampus [38, 39]; antagonism of

5-HT2A, 5-HT2C or 5-HT6 receptors [40] and stimulation of 5-HT1A receptors [41]. An increased release of DA may particularly lead to stimulation of D1 and D3 receptors, with a possibly beneficial effect on cognition, assuming that these receptors are under-stimulated in schizophrenia [39]. An increased release of Ach might lead to enhancement of M1, M4, or α7 nicotinic acid postsynaptic receptors, all of which have been indicated as potentially involved in cognitive impairment in schizophrenia [42]. However, cognitive improvements observed with SGAs may reflect avoidance of potentially deleterious effects associated with FGAs rather than a specific enhancement of cognition [43]. About SGAs, specific effects of each drug on the cognitive function are shown in Table 2.1. A meta-analysis by Woodward et al. [55] demonstrated that SGAs improved overall cognitive function to a greater extent than FGAs. McGurk et al. [60] demonstrated a significant improvement in several cognitive domains (selective attention, executive functioning, verbal learning and memory, and verbal fluency) in partial responders to FGAs antipsychotics who had been switched to olanzapine. Furthermore, Wang et al. [61] reported that olanzapine could significantly improve short-term memory, immediate memory, and memory quotient in first-episode schizophrenic patients. Some findings suggest that aripiprazole may offer advantages over olanzapine in improving neurocognitive function [62]. In an independent systematic review, Houthoofd et al. [63] reported positive effects of risperidone on neurocognitive function in patients with schizophrenia and schizoaffective disorder in processing speed, attention/vigilance, verbal and visual learning, and memory and in reasoning and problem solving. However, the effect of risperidone on social cognition in patients with schizophrenia remains controversial due to conflicting results [64]. Amisulpride seems to improve verbal fluency performance, attention, and working memory [45, 46], with particular benefits on this last one when associated with aripiprazole [65]. Clozapine improves significantly attention and verbal fluency, but only modestly executive functioning and delayed recall [54, 55]. Carpenter and Gold [43] reported small advantages of SGAs compared to FGAs in terms of cognitive performance. As shown above, the studies that have focused on the possible differential effects of specific SGAs were not conclusive. In this regard, although a meta-analysis on SGAs effect on cognitive functioning in patients with schizophrenia was able to detect some interesting preliminary results, these were mostly controversial, not showing any uniform effect of each SGAs on cognitive profile [66]. Moreover, a recent meta-analysis on the effect of SGAs subcategories on the cognitive profile of patients with schizophrenia, based upon the chemical structure (the *-pines* and the *-dones*), showed that the cognitive effect of the two SGAs categories was overall comparable (significant, with a small ES), and there were no clear evidence that the pattern of cognitive effects was different between the two SGAs subtype [67].

On the other hand, given that individual SGAs show different pharmacological profiles and that cognitive function consists of different domains, it is possible that the effects on cognitive function may differ among drugs. This is in line with results from a network meta-analysis study that found SGAs' different effects on distinct cognitive domains in schizophrenia patients. In particular, quetiapine, risperidone, and olanzapine had better effects on the overall cognitive profile than amisulpride

Table 2.1 Mechanism of action and effects of antipsychotic agents on cognitive profile in schizophrenia

Agent	Mechanism of action [44]	Effects on cognition
Amisulpride	Dopamine D2R (putatively with regional selectivity)	Improvement in verbal fluency performance, attention, frontal dysfunction, and working memory [45, 46]
Aripiprazole	Partial dopamine D2R agonism (>serotonin 5HT1A partial agonism ≥ serotonin 5HT2A)	Improvements in reaction time and in attention with correct responses to stimuli and in cognitive functioning [39, 47, 48]
Asenapine	High affinity for 5HT1A, 5HT1B, 5HT2A, 5HT2C, 5HT6 and 5HT7, and among DA receptors (higher for D3R than D2R). D1R activation	Improve processing speed, verbal learning, and memory compared to placebo [39, 49]
Brexpiprazole	Partial agonist at 5-HT1A and D2R at similar potencies and antagonist at 5-HT2A and adrenergic alpha1B/2C receptors. Less intrinsic agonist activity at D2R than aripiprazole	Significant benefit on measures of psychosocial, occupational, and cognitive functioning, particularly attention/vigilance and visual learning [50, 51]
Cariprazine	Partial agonist of D3R, D2R, 5HT1A; antagonist of 5HT2A, 5HT2A, 5HT2C, 5HT7. Higher affinity for D3R, than aripiprazole and brexpiprazole	It may be effective in treating negative symptoms and several aspects of cognition associated with schizophrenia, such as recognition memory and rule learning [39, 52, 53]
Clozapine	Cholinergic M1 > serotonin 5HT2A > histamine H1 > serotonin 5HT2C > alpha 1 > alpha 2 ≫> D2R	Great improvements in attention and verbal fluency, but modest benefits about executive functioning and delayed recall [39, 54, 55]
Lurasidone	Strong antagonist of D2R, 5-HT2A, and 5HT7, partial agonist of 5HT1A and partial antagonist of α2C [56]	Great improvements in speed of processing domain at 160 mg/die; improvements in visual learning, working memory, reasoning/problem solving, and social cognition at 40/80 or 120 mg/day [50, 57]
Olanzapine	Histamine H1 > serotonin 5HT2A > cholinergic M1 > serotonin 5HT2C > dopamine D2R	Great improvements in vigilance, selective attention, delayed recall, verbal learning and memory, verbal fluency, and executive functioning [54, 55]
Paliperidone	Serotonin 5HT2A > dopamine D2R	Paliperidone ER was more beneficial in the improvement of verbal memory and social function compared with risperidone [58]
Quetiapine	Alpha 1 > histamine H1 > serotonin 5HT2A > alpha 2 > cholinergic H1 ≫ dopamine D2R; SRI	Improvements on global cognitive functioning in the early stage of treatment and verbal short-term memory [59]
Risperidone	Serotonin 5HT2A ≫ alpha 1 > dopamine D2R	Moderate improvements in working memory, executive functioning, attention, and delayed recall [39, 54, 55]

DA dopamine, *5-HT* 5-hydroxytryptamine (serotonin), *mPFC* medial prefrontal cortex, *SRI* serotonin reuptake inhibition and haloperidol, but when a single cognitive domain was considered, quetiapine, risperidone, and olanzapine were better than amisulpride on executive functions, quetiapine was better than other antipsychotics on attention and processing speed, followed by ziprasidone and olanzapine, and ziprasidone was better than amisulpride and haloperidol on memory [68].

Lastly, treatment with antipsychotic medication is associated with moderate improvement in cognitive performance among patients with schizophreniform disorder and in patients at their first episode of psychosis (FEP) [61, 68, 69].

2.2.4 Cognitive Functioning in Schizophrenia: Focus on Long-Acting Injectable (LAI) Antipsychotics

Several studies observed an improvement in the cognitive functioning by switching from oral formulation of antipsychotics to a long-acting injectable (LAI) formulation. For example, switching from oral risperidone to risperidone LAI (R-LAI) seems to improve verbal memory [70], with a significantly greater mean changes from baseline on the STM-COMET memory scanning test and memory filtering test. Switching from oral risperidone to R-LAI may affect motor processing function and attention improvement efficacy by allowing the dosage of anti-Parkinson's medications (such as biperiden and an anticholinergic drug) to be reduced. The benefits of switching from an oral therapy to a LAI one are also shown in another study, where patients who switched from oral risperidone to paliperidone LAI showed greater improvements in attention and processing speed compared to those who continued on risperidone [71].

As for the oral formulation, second-generation LAI appears to be better on the cognitive profile also if compared to the first-generation LAI. For example, comparing Haloperidol Decanoas with R-LAI, patients whose therapy was switched to second-generation LAI exhibited significant improvement in memory, executive function, motor processing function, and attention. Also in these cases, a possible explanation could be that FGAs determine EPS more often than SGAs [72, 73] and, for this reason, their use can lead to the coadministration of anti-Parkinson's medications; this association is known to result in cognitive dysfunction [74, 75]. These observations seem confirmed also in the comparison between first- and other second-generation LAI: for example, switching to aripiprazole LAI seems to be associated with a better cognitive function in verbal memory, working memory, verbal fluency, and executive function [76].

2.2.5 Cognitive Functioning in Schizophrenia: Focus on Antidepressants

In major depressive disorder (MDD), antidepressants are generally associated with beneficial effects on cognitive impairment, which may be mediated at least in part by the improvement obtained in affective symptoms, making it a partially indirect effect [77]. Interventions targeting multiple neurochemical systems simultaneously (e.g., serotonin-norepinephrine reuptake inhibitor, SNRIs, such as duloxetine) might be more likely to improve cognitive performance than treatments targeting only a single system (e.g., selective serotonin reuptake inhibitor, SSRIs, such as escitalopram) [78]. Furthermore, vortioxetine seems to improve cognitive symptoms in major depressive disorder (MDD) through its multimodal action, in particular on different serotoninergic receptors which may modulate glutamatergic neurotransmission [79, 80]. For these reasons, several clinical studies have evaluated the effects of antidepressants on cognitive performance in schizophrenia. In preliminary studies, SSRIs seem not to have any effects on cognitive functions [81], while bupropion, a noradrenaline and dopamine reuptake inhibitor, showed an improvement in attention tests [82]. Moreover, mirtazapine seems to improve visual-spatial ability and general mental speed/attentional control [83] and mianserin added to FGAs showed improvements on memory and learning skills [84]. Unfortunately, a meta-analysis which evaluates the effect of antidepressant augmentation of antipsychotics for the treatment of cognitive deficits in schizophrenia, found no clinically meaningful improvement in any cognitive domain or the composite score [85]. These findings suggest that, in patients with chronic schizophrenia, cognition does not appear to be significantly improved by the enhancement of serotonergic or noradrenergic neurotransmission on top of antipsychotic. However, antidepressants have been found in some studies to significantly reduce negative symptoms [86–90], but also depressive symptoms in schizophrenia patients with comorbid MDD [91].

2.2.6 Cognitive Functioning in Schizophrenia: Focus on New Pharmacological Targets

The exact mechanism of cognitive dysfunction in schizophrenia is still debated, but the most supported hypotheses are the glutamatergic, cholinergic, GABAergic, and histaminergic ones [92, 93]. Consequently, a number of GABAergic agents have been studied to stimulate cognition in schizophrenia. Precisely, a dysfunction of γ-aminobutyric acid (GABA) interneurons has been suggested in the pathophysiology of schizophrenia, as the result of a reduction of GABA interneuron density in the frontal cortex and, consequently, an imbalance between excitation and inhibition in the cerebral cortex [94]. According to the "GABA hypofunction" theory [95], a developmental deficit of inhibitory GABA interneurons may underlie neurodegeneration through an excessive activation of glutamatergic neurons [96]. Moreover, an imbalance between excitatory and inhibitory (E-I) activity, induced by a low activity of glutamatergic projections and GABA interneurons in the prefrontal cortex, may lead to impaired working memory in schizophrenia [97]. To correct the "E-I imbalance," new compounds have been developed to treat negative symptoms and cognitive deficits [98], as the agonists of the glycine site of NMDA receptor, DA-D1 receptor, metabotropic glutamate receptor, and 5-HT1A receptors [99]. Clinical evidence suggests that serotonin 5-HT1A receptor agonists improve cognitive deficits in schizophrenia, through the correction of the E-I imbalance via the suppression of GABA neural function [100]. Several compounds have been developed to influence GABA activity, but most of these compounds have failed to demonstrate neurocognitive benefits in large clinical trials [101].

The effects of glutamatergic agents on cognitive deficits have also been investigated. Glutamate is the major excitatory neurotransmitter in the central nervous system and its receptors include NMDA and AMPA receptors. NMDA receptor antagonists, such as ketamine and phencyclidine, can produce clinical and cognitive symptoms of schizophrenia in healthy individuals, leading to the hypothesis that the NMDA receptor could be involved in the pathophysiology of psychosis [102]. Several clinical trials have examined the neurocognitive enhancement benefits of a group of amino acids that act as glutamate agonists by binding to the glycine site on NMDA receptors. These NMDA receptor agonists include glycine, D-cycloserine, and D-serine but none of the currently published studies produced evidence about their benefits on neurocognition: in an initial exploratory study, a single dose of D-cycloserine improved performance on a delayed recall task, but later studies were not able to replicate this finding. Conversely, glycine has shown a beneficial effect as an adjunctive agent to antipsychotics for negative and cognitive symptoms [103].

Cholinergic agents act on the central cholinergic system, which innervates a diverse range of cortical and subcortical structures, interacting through coordinated acetylcholine (ACh) release with nicotinic and muscarinic receptors [104]. The once common practice of co-administering anticholinergic and antimuscarinic agents to schizophrenic patients treated with FGAs to reduce EPS side effects, used to determine a worsening in cognitive impairments [105]. In healthy subjects, the acute administration of antimuscarinic agents can produce cognitive impairments that mimic the deficits observed in schizophrenic patients [106]. Significant reductions in the expression of M1 and M4 receptors have been consistently reported in the postmortem brains of schizophrenic patients in regions linked to cognitive function, including the hippocampus, frontal and prefrontal cortex, superior temporal gyrus, and the anterior and posterior cingulate cortex [107]. Conversely, the expressions of M2 and M3 receptors have been reported as unaltered in the brains of patients with schizophrenia across a number of cortical regions [108]. In accordance with this evidence, it has been suggested that a dysfunctional muscarinic system is contributing to the symptoms of schizophrenia and might represent a therapeutic target [109]. In this regard, clozapine was the first atypical antipsychotic to show nootropic attributes inducing mild improvements across a number of cognitive functions, including learning and memory [110], eventually attributed to its effects on the muscarinic system. Galantamine is a competitive and reversible cholinesterase inhibitor that also acts as an M1 muscarinic acetylcholine receptor agonist or a modulator of $\alpha 4$ and $\alpha 7$ nicotinic receptors, and has been used primarily in the treatment of early stage of vascular dementia and Alzheimer's disease [111]: this drug produced neurocognitive benefits in schizophrenic patients [112, 113]. The five muscarinic receptors share considerable orthosteric binding site homogeneity, while they present a secondary allosteric binding site, which is substantially heterogeneous and became the target for most recently developed drugs. Positive allosteric modulators (PAMs) are a class of allosteric agonists that increase the receptor's affinity for ACh at the orthosteric binding site and consequentially potentiate the receptor's response to Ach [114]. BQCA [115] and PQCA [116] are strong, highly selective M1 receptor PAM reported to produce pro-cognitive responses, including enhancing memory function and increasing spontaneous prefrontal brain activity in preclinical trials. In addition to antipsychotic-like qualities, the M4 receptor PAM, VU0467154 [117], and VU1052100 [118] have been reported to enhance cognition. However, more investigations are required to determine the suitability of muscarinic PAMs as new treatments against psychotic and cognitive symptoms in schizophrenia patients.

Development strategies of nicotinic agents mostly focused on the α7-subtype of the nicotinic acetylcholine receptor because of a variety of factors: the genetic links between this subunit and schizophrenia, its high expression rates in key cognitive processing areas (e.g., hippocampus, thalamus, and prefrontal cortex) and the evidence of a decreased expression in postmortem studies on patients' brains [119]. The α7 nicotinic acetylcholine receptors (α7 receptors) have been shown to play an important role in cognition and have potential therapeutic applications in cognitive impairment in schizophrenia as well as in Alzheimer's disease [120]. Encenicline demonstrated clinically meaningful improvements in cognition and functioning in patients with schizophrenia, whereas varenicline, an α7-subtype of the nicotinic acetylcholine receptor agonist originally approved for smoking cessation, and tropisetron, a 5-HT3 receptor antagonist and α7-subtype of the nicotinic Ach receptor partial agonist approved as antiemetic agent, showed the same inconsistent effects on cognition in schizophrenia [121]. Several cognitive enhancers approved for Alzheimer's Disease, such as antidementia agents (donepezil, rivastigmine, galantamine, and memantine), have been tested for their potential to improve cognition in schizophrenia. Unfortunately, cognitive deficits in schizophrenia and in Alzheimer's disease are determined by different mechanisms, as recent findings suggest [122]. Studies on the acetylcholinesterase inhibitors, such as donepezil, rivastigmine, and galantamine, gave mixed [123] or negative results [124] in schizophrenia patients. Memantine, usually prescribed as neurocognitive enhancer in Alzheimer's disease, has several mechanisms of action. Although memantine may have possible procognitive effects in schizophrenia patients [125], it does not appear to produce any benefit when added to atypical antipsychotic therapy [126, 127].

Oxytocin is a hypothalamic peptide contributing to maternal–infant bonding. Several smaller studies were done evaluating the effects on social cognitive functioning of this molecule administered intranasally in people with schizophrenia. Further testing is needed to explain whether oxytocin has therapeutic potential for social cognitive deficits and/or negative symptoms in schizophrenic patients [128].

Guanfacine, atomoxetine, and reboxetine, three noradrenergic compounds, have been evaluated for their hypothetical procognitive benefits in people with schizophrenia; however, in published clinical trials, all of them have demonstrated a lack of efficacy in this population [129–131].

Some published studies on serotoninergic agents have evaluated tandospirone [132], buspirone [133], and ondansetron [134]. However, no study has suggested robust procognitive effects of these compounds.

Following the hypothesis that inflammation plays a role in the pathogenesis of schizophrenia, several drugs targeting neuroinflammation and oxidative stress were studied. In fact, increased rates of schizophrenia were observed after infectious events, such as maternal exposure to flu and upper respiratory infections. Studies revealed that in pregnant women, an augmented expression of inflammatory cytokines in the second trimester increased the risk of schizophrenia in their offspring [135]. Viral exposure can reduce the density of receptors relevant for neurocognition, such as D1 receptors in the frontal areas and NMDA receptors in the hippocampus, it can decrease protein kinase B expression and impair axonal integrity [136]. Levels of proinflammatory cytokines, such as interleukin IL-6, are elevated in schizophrenia [137] and have been shown to influence specific brain regions, including prefrontal cortex, medial temporal regions, and long-term potentiation in the hippocampus [138]. IL-6 increases oxidative stress, which may interfere with the expression of inhibitory GABA interneurons and impact executive functioning [139]: levels of C-reactive protein (CRP), an inflammatory biomarker, are associated with neurocognitive deficits, but not necessarily with symptom severity in people with schizophrenia [140]. Neuroinflammation indirectly slows neurogenesis, synaptogenesis, and dendritic growth as it impacts the activity-dependent transport of brain-derived neurotrophic factor (BDNF), a neuroplasticity-regulating protein [141]. Given their impact on neurocognition, neuroinflammation and oxidative stress are potential targets for psychopharmacological enhancement of neurocognition. Minocycline, a broad-spectrum antibiotic, is a long-acting tetracycline traditionally prescribed for the treatment of bacterial infections. There has been recent interest about possible anti-inflammatory, anti-oxidative, and neuroprotective benefits of minocycline in people with neurodegenerative disorders and in people with schizophrenia [142]. In this context, also acetylsalicylic acid (aspirin), traditionally used as an analgesic and an antipyretic medication, has gained recent interest as an anti-inflammatory agent in schizophrenia [142]. Particular attention has been paid to the anti-inflammatory properties of simvastatin and rosuvastatin; however, evidences are sparse [143].

Also, interest emerged about the possible procognitive effect of modafinil, a stimulant drug marked as a "wakefulness-promoting medication," that has a yet unclear mechanism of action, but it appears to show therapeutic effects by increasing the expression of histamine in the hypothalamus [144]. Modafinil activates glutamatergic circuits while inhibiting GABA and seems to act as a dopamine agonist, inhibiting the reuptake of dopamine by binding to the dopamine reuptake transporter [145]. In some studies, modafinil was shown to improve attention, memory and executive functioning in people with schizophrenia [146]; however, several studies found no benefits of this agent [147, 148].

Omega-3 fatty acids are known to be essential for normal cortical expansion and maturation and functional integrity during prenatal and postnatal phases and during adult development [149]. It has been demonstrated that omega-3 fatty acids may be beneficial to decrease the risk of a frank psychotic disorder in ultra-high-risk individuals, suggesting possible neuroprotective effects [150]. However, very few clinical studies on omega-3 fatty acids have examined their neurocognitive benefits.

Some studies demonstrated that the adjunctive use of *N*-acetylcysteine, a precursor of glutathione with antioxidant effects, improved the negative symptoms of schizophrenia, although there was no direct examination of its neurocognitive benefits [151].

Cannabis sativa is the most widely used drug in the world. It contains over 70 different constituents, including delta-9-tetrahydrocannabinol (Δ9-THC) and cannabidiol (CBD) [152]. CBD can interfere with the detrimental actions of Δ9-THC in terms of psychotic proneness and cognitive dysfunction [153]. On the other hand, CBD is a particularly interesting target as a novel approach for cognitive improvement in schizophrenia, in part, due to its strong anti-inflammatory properties [154]. CBD has the potential to limit Δ9THC-induced cognitive impairment and to improve cognitive function in different pathological conditions, but there is limited evidence investigating the therapeutic efficacy of CBD as treatment for cognitive deficits in schizophrenia [155, 156]. However, evidences suggesting cognitive improvement in neurological disorders with CBD treatment emerged [157].

The main characteristics of the new drugs described above are shown in Table 2.2.

Table 2.2 Mechanism of action and effects of the new pharmacological targets on cognitive profile in schizophrenia

Category/agent		Mechanism of action	Effect
NMDA agents [158–161]	Glycine	Co-agonist at glycine site	Added to antipsychotics, it is associated with some benefits in negative and cognitive symptoms
	D-cycloserine	Co-agonist at glycine site and partial agonist	Lack of procognitive efficacy
	D-serine	Co-agonist at glycine site	Lack of procognitive efficacy
AMPA-R agents [159, 160]	AMPA-R agonists	Possible positive allosteric modulating activity at AMPA-R (i.e., act as "AMPA-kines")	Improve in Working Memory, with a small positive effect

(continued)

Table 2.2 (continued)

Category/agent		Mechanism of action	Effect
Cholinergic agents [159–162]	Encenicline	α7 nAChR partial agonist	Some improvements in cognition and functioning
	Varencicline	α7 nAChR full agonist	Lack/poor procognitive efficacy
	Tropisetron	α7 nAChR partial agonist and 5HT3 receptor antagonist	Lack/poor procognitive efficacy
Anti-dementia agents [159–161]	Donepezil	Acetylcholinesterase inhibitor, increasing concentration of Ach at the synapse	Lack of procognitive efficacy
	Rivastigmine	Acetylcholinesterase inhibitor, increasing concentration of Ach at the synapse	Lack of procognitive efficacy
	Galantamine	Acetylcholinesterase inhibitor as well as nicotinic receptor agonist	Lack/poor procognitive efficacy
	Memantine	NMDA receptor antagonist	Poor procognitive efficacy
Hypothalamic peptide [128, 160]	Oxytocin	It contributes to maternal–infant bonding	Effects on social cognitive deficits and/or negative symptoms
Noradrenergic agents [159]	Guanfacine	α2 adrenergic agonist	Lack of procognitive efficacy
	Atomoxetine	Selective inhibition of presynaptic norepinephrine reuptake	Poor procognitive efficacy
	Reboxetine	Selective norepinephrine reuptake inhibitor	Lack of procognitive efficacy
Serotoninergic agents [163, 164]	Tandospirone	5-HT1A receptor partial agonist	Lack of robust procognitive effect
	Buspirone	High affinity for 5-HT1A and 5-HT2 receptors	Lack of robust procognitive effect
	Ondansetron	Selective 5-HT3 receptor antagonist	Lack of robust procognitive effect

Table 2.2 (continued)

Category/agent		Mechanism of action	Effect
Anti-inflammatory agents [160, 165]	Minocycline	Broad-spectrum tetracycline antibiotic with anti-inflammatory and anti-apoptotic properties	Some procognitive efficacy in add-on with antipsychotics
	Acetylsalicylic acid	Anti-inflammatory agent with analgesic and antipyretic properties	Lack of procognitive efficacy
	Simvastatin	Used for prevention of cardiovascular disease and for treatment of abnormal lipids, presented anti-inflammatory properties	Lack of procognitive efficacy
	Rosuvastatin	Used for prevention of cardiovascular disease and for treatment of abnormal lipids, presented anti-inflammatory properties	Lack of procognitive efficacy
Stimulant agents [146, 159]	Modafinil	It stimulates histamine, norepinephrine, serotonin, dopamine, and orexin and reduces GABA release	Lack of efficacy/some procognitive effects in early schizophrenia
Other agents [25, 157, 165–167]	Omega-3 fatty acids	Regulate normal cortical expansion and maturation and functional integrity during prenatal and postnatal phases and during adult development	Poor efficacy/some procognitive efficacy in schizophrenic patients with metabolic syndrome
	N-acetylcysteine	Precursor of glutathione with antioxidant effects	Controversial efficacy/potential effect on working memory
	Cannabis sativa	Its constituent, known as cannabidiol, presented strong anti-inflammatory properties	Lack/poor procognitive efficacy

AMPA-R α-amino-3-hydroxy-5-methyl-4-isoxazolepropionic acid receptor, *GABA* γ-aminobutyric acid, *5-HT* 5-hydroxytryptamine (serotonin), *nAChR* nicotinic acetylcholine receptor, *NMDA* *N*-methyl-D-aspartate

2.3 Non-pharmacological Interventions to Improve Cognitive Functioning in Schizophrenia: Focus on Cognitive Remediation

New non-pharmacological interventions to improve cognitive symptoms in schizophrenia are under study, with the ultimate goal to also obtain a better functional outcome [168]. These interventions, including cognitive remediation (CR) approaches, are enclosed in a positive light and they are grounded in a recovery rather than a deficit model [126, 127]. This new interest is based on the factors associated with an improved quality of life, such as the ability to enjoy social and familial interactions, the advance in educational endeavors and performing well at work. The underlying theoretical framework of these improvements comes from the modern neuroscientific knowledge, which supports the idea that brain would be able of changes and development throughout lifespan [169]. According to this perspective, psychosocial interventions base their theoretical principles on the concept of cerebral plasticity and neurogenesis [17, 170]. As stated by different scientific theories, the development of skills can occur at any age and can help to advance or to restore the brain capacity for improving cognitive and social performance [169]. Learning in an appropriately stimulating environment can help the patient to benefit from brain malleability and to improve functioning [171]. In the next paragraph, we will present a definition of CR interventions and their general principles and features. Then we will review the main results reported in recent meta-analyses regarding the efficacy of CR treatments in experimental conditions as well as their effectiveness "in the real world," underlining also the potential neurobiological correlates of the effects of CR in patients with schizophrenia. We will also review current evidence of possible benefits deriving from CR in the early course of schizophrenia and in subjects "at risk" of psychosis.

2.4 What Is Cognitive Remediation and How Does It Work?

One of the first definitions of CR was "the therapeutic process of increasing or improving an individual's capacity to process and use incoming information in order to allow increased functioning in everyday life." This includes methods to train and restore cognitive function and compensatory techniques [172]. More recently, during Cognitive Remediation Experts Workshop (CREW), the definition of CR for schizophrenia became "a behavioural training-based intervention that aims to improve cognitive processes (attention, memory, executive functions, social cognition or metacognition) with the goal of durability and generalization." According to those experts, "the effectiveness of this training is enhanced when provided in a context (formal or informal) that gives support and opportunity for extending everyday functioning" (Florence 2010). As mentioned above, CR bases its theoretical principles on the concept of cerebral plasticity and neurogenesis [170]. Sure enough this intervention, when carried out in a stimulating context, seems to facilitate the development of brain plasticity [171]. CR strategies can be distinguished into two main models: compensatory and restorative [173]. The treatments based on compensatory strategies try to bypass or to eliminate the specific cognitive deficit, using the subject residual cognitive abilities. On the other hand, the restorative methods use the capacity of the brain to develop and repair itself throughout lifetime; these strategies are based on knowledge about neuronal plasticity, working with the aim to correct a specific deficit by repairing the specific underlying compromised function. Furthermore, restorative remediation strategies utilize two different approaches: bottom-up and top-down [174]. Bottom-up approaches start with the remediation of basic neurocognitive skills (e.g., attention) and advance to more complex skills (e.g., problem solving). Quite the opposite, top-down approaches use more complex skills with the aim to enhance single and specific neurocognitive domains. Therefore, some restorative strategies take advantage of the use of drill and practice exercises in order to restore cognitive functions and, possibly, to improve neuronal plasticity. On the other hand, other techniques are based on the implementation of new strategies and tend to favor the generalization in different contexts through the execution of different tasks that involve the use of similar strategies [173]. In this context, some CR programs focus on a specific cognitive deficit (e.g., attention or ToM), whereas others work on multiple cognitive domains and are more comprehensive. It is undoubtedly possible that all the above-mentioned CR strategies would be complementary and synergic and that the potentiation of specific target functions may favor the development of new compensatory strategies of problem solving, which could be applied and could influence the patient's daily life [15, 175, 176]. CR techniques can be advocated as a package that provides a standard set of exercises or it may be personalized only to target deficits identified in a single individual [177]. To reach the established objectives, CR employs several learning strategies: errorless learning, scaffolding, positive reinforcement, massed practice, and information processing strategies [175]. Errorless learning inhibits the implicit encoding of errors, which cannot then be differentiated from correct information by explicit recall. Scaffolding is similar to errorless learning in ensuring a high degree of success for the learner and minimizing errors, by carefully regulating the complexity of the material to be learnt. The trainee is encouraged to use previously established areas of competence, while help is provided with new aspects of learning. Massed practice consists in the practice of repeated exercise (at least 2–3 times per week) in order to encourage the upkeep and application of the skills developed. Information processing strategies involve verbalization, information reduction, breaking and simplifying the task into smaller steps, providing written prompts, chunking, self-monitoring, mnemonic strategies, categorization, organization, and planning. These strategies are otherwise applied to various levels in different methods of CR, depending on whether they are primarily based on repeated execution of specific tasks or on the implementation of new strategies [173]. A few factors influence a positive treatment response for CR training, such as training of the therapist, motivation of the patient, type and intensity of training, and cognitive resources at baseline [15]. In past decades, a number of CR techniques have been developed and adopted in multimodal treatment approaches in schizophrenia: computerized and noncomputerized, designed for individual or group settings. The main structured protocols of cognitive training for schizophrenia are described in Table 2.3. At the same time, many authors investigated the efficacy on CR in patients with schizophrenia. In the next paragraph, we will analyze the principal results about this topic.

Table 2.3 The main structured cognitive remediation protocols in schizophrenia

Cognitive training	Target	Duration	Setting (individual/group)	Computer assisted/not computer assisted	Restorative/compensatory	Top-down	Bottom-up	Drill and practice	Strategy coaching	Individual adjustment
IPT [178]	Cognitive functions, social skills, and problem solving	Sessions of 60 min, 2–3 times a week (about 12 months)	Group (6–8)	Not computer assisted	Restorative	+	+	+	+	–
CRT [176]	Cognitive functions	40 sessions at least 3 times a week, 45–60 min each one	Individual	Not computer-assisted session	Restorative	+	+	+	+	+
NET [179]	Cognitive functions and social cognition	Sessions of 45 min at least 5 times a week (about 6 months)	Individual/group	Computer-assisted sessions and not computer-assisted sessions	Restorative	–	+	+	–	+
NEAR [180]	Cognitive functions and problem solving	Sessions of 60 min, twice a week (about 4 months)	Individual/group (3–10)	Computer-assisted sessions and not computer-assisted sessions	Restorative	+	–	–	+	+

CET [181]	Cognitive functions and social cognition	Biweekly sessions (about 2.5 h every week) for 24 months	Group (couples and then groups of 3–4 couples)	Computer-assisted sessions and not computer-assisted sessions	Restorative	+	+	+	+	–
INT [182]	Cognitive functions and social cognition	30 biweekly sessions, 90 min each one	Group (6–8)	Computer-assisted sessions and not computer-assisted sessions	Restorative	+	+	+	+	–
SSANIT [183]	Cognitive functions, social cognition and social skills	NT: biweekly sessions of 1 h SST: weekly sessions of 2 h Duration: 6 months	Individual (group)	NT sessions: computer-assisted SST sessions: not computer assisted	Restorative	+	+	+	+	+
TAR [184]	Social cognition	12 sessions twice a week, 45 min each one	Small groups of two patients and a psychotherapist	Computer-assisted sessions and not computer-assisted sessions	Restorative/ compensatory	–	+	+	+	+
SCIT [185]	Social cognition	24 weekly sessions, 50 min each one (about 6 months)	Group (6–8)	Computer-assisted sessions and not computer-assisted group sessions	Restorative	–	+	+	+	–

(continued)

Table 2.3 (continued)

Cognitive training	Target	Duration	Setting (individual/group)	Computer assisted/not computer assisted	Restorative/compensatory	Top-down	Bottom-up	Drill and practice	Strategy coaching	Individual adjustment
SCET [186]	Social cognition, ToM	36 sessions of 90 min, twice a week (about 6 months)	Group	Not computer assisted	Restorative	–	+	+	+	–
SCST [187]	Social cognition	12 weekly sessions, 60 min each one (about 3 months)	Group (6 patients)	Computer-assisted sessions and not computer-assisted group sessions	Restorative	–	+	+	+	–
Cogpack[a] (CACR)	Cognitive functions	Sessions variables in duration and frequency (starting from 2 to 3 weeks)	Individual	Computer assisted	Restorative	–	+	+	–	+
CIRCUITS [188]	Cognitive functions and metacognition	12 sessions, three times a week, 60 min each one (40 sessions)	Individual	Web-based computerized CR therapy with therapist plus independent session	Restorative	+	+	+	+	+

CCT [189]	Cognitive functions	12 two hour-weekly sessions, (about 3 months)	Group (4–8 patients)	Group sessions with two facilitators	Compensatory	+	+	+	+	–

CCT compensatory cognitive training, *CET* cognitive enhancement therapy, *CRT* cognitive remediation therapy, *INT* integrated neurocognitive therapy, *IPT* integrated psychological therapy, *MCT* metacognitive training, *NEAR* neuropsychological educational approach to remediation, *NET* neurocognitive enhancement therapy, *NT* neurocognitive training, *SCET* social cognition enhancement training, *SCIT* social cognition and interaction training, *SCST* social cognitive skills training, *SSANIT* social skills and neurocognitive individualized training, *SST* social skills training, *TAR* training of affect recognition, *ToM* theory of mind

[a] Cogpack (www.markersoftware.com) is a typical computer-assisted cognitive remediation (CACR) technique

2.5 Cognitive Remediation: Focus on Social and Nonsocial Cognition

Starting from the definition of CR, we know that one of the aims of these behavioral training-based interventions is to improve cognitive processes, which are recognized as the most important predictors of functional outcome and quality of life in people with schizophrenia [190]. Various published meta-analyses support the efficacy of CR for enhancing cognitive outcomes. Nevertheless, the first results that we can find from the literature are controversial. In two independent reviews, Kurtz et al. [191] and Twamley et al. [192] underlined that CR programs have effective components that hold promise for improving cognitive performance (with a medium or large ES). On the other hand Pilling et al. [193], in a first review based on a few studies, reported that CR had no benefit on attention, verbal memory, visual memory, planning, cognitive flexibility, or mental state and concluded that CR did not appear to confer reliable benefits for patients with schizophrenia and could not be recommended for clinical practice. After the earliest reviews, it was developed a rich body of literature that well established that CR is effective in reducing cognitive deficits with long-term benefits in schizophrenia [19, 191, 192, 194–198]. All these reviews find a moderate ES of CR programs in improving neurocognitive deficit. The results about cognition acquire robustness when CR is associated with psychiatric rehabilitation: this combination led to significant favorable outcomes for global cognition [196, 199]. One of the most important meta-analyses of the available controlled studies of CR in schizophrenia performed by Wykes et al. [19] including 40 studies and about 2000 patients, showed a moderate improvement in overall cognitive performance (more effective when patients were clinically stable). Authors declare that no treatment element (remediation approach, duration, computer use, etc.) was associated with cognitive outcome. This work underlined some durability of the effects (ES = 0.43), as shown in follow-up studies [200]. Durability of effects was also underlined in a recent study performed by Buonocore et al. [201], who found out that all cognitive abilities improved with CR, in association with standard rehabilitation, remained stable over time from the end of treatment to evaluation at 5 years, except for psychomotor speed and coordination that showed a significant decrease. Positive effects of CR on global cognition were found also in a recent metanalytic work, indicating that CR improves cognition across several domains including processing speed, working memory, and learning, much more in inpatient settings [202]. Overall, the most recent and comprehensive meta-analysis on the effectiveness of CR for people living with schizophrenia included 130 studies and a total of 8.851 participants, found a consistent small-to-moderate positive effect of CR on social and nonsocial cognitive performance [203].

Regarding the instrument utilized to administer CR, computer-assisted cognitive remediation (CACR) methods [204] showed significant improvement, especially on the domains of attention and working memory (marginally on other neurocognitive domains). Moreover, a recent meta-analytic study performed by Kambeitz-Ilankovic et al. [205] underlined that the effects of CR on cognitive outcomes are consistently reported both for training administered in a computerized fashion and for training supplemented by human guidance (SHG). Nonetheless, the comparison between CR administered with or without human guidance revealed that the human approach gives largest effects on the cognitive subdomains of working and verbal memory. On the other hand, no difference was reported between individual and group methods.

A substantial but controversial body of literature was presented also for social cognition, starting from the first meta-analysis that debates this topic, performed by Grynszpan et al. [194], highlighting the efficacy of CACR, particularly in social cognition and ending with some specific reviews that analyze promising results of training specifically developed for social cognition in schizophrenia. For example, a meta-analysis performed by Kurtz and Richardson [195] stressed the greatest effect of social cognitive treatments on facial affect recognition (FAR), with a moderate-to-large ES for affect identification and a large ES for affect discrimination. Authors also reported a moderate ES for ToM and a large impact on measures of observer-rated community and institutional functioning. According to Yeh et al. [206], that more recently conduct a meta-analytic work on CACR and social cognition with particular attention regarding ToM, there are different recent results around this topic. Prikken and colleagues in fact [204] found no effect of CACR on social cognition, whereas Lindenmayer et al. [207] suggested that CACR could enhance social cognition. Authors highlight that findings are inconsistent also regarding the relationship between ToM deficits and cognitive load in schizophrenia [208–211]. Hence, they focused their analysis on CACR and ToM in schizophrenia, founding that computerized training did not significantly enhance affective ToM ($p = 0.42$), instead treatments without computerized training were significantly superior in terms of improving cognitive ToM.

Concerning all different methods of interventions (CACR and pen and pencil), two recent systematic reviews [212, 213] highlight positive results, emphasizing that targeted interventions produce more significant improvements, particularly in the domains of affect recognition, emotion processing and ToM. Results were less clear for social perception, a complex construct that tends to be culturally specific [214], and for attributional bias, domains that appear to be more difficult to measure and train. Such skill in "cognitive restructuring" is thus more challenging for people with schizophrenia to acquire, compared to emotion perception training which comprises drills and practice to achieve implicit learning and automation [215, 216].

Promising results were found also in a recent meta-analysis performed by Nijman et al. [217] that investigate the efficacy and the durability of different types of social cognition training, with an analysis of moderators of treatment outcome. Authors found that broad-based social cognition training significantly improved emotion perception, social perception, ToM, and social functioning. Targeted social cognition training had the largest effect on emotion perception and social perception. These improvements were maintained at follow-up but were generally less than at post-treatment. Regarding treatment variables that significantly moderated outcome, they underlined that individual treatments were more effective for emotion perception, but group treatments worked better to improve social functioning.

In recent years, studies about CR pay their attention to a better understanding of whom is able to benefit from CR: this knowledge would enable clinicians to more effectively refer patients to CR or tailor the intervention to the individual [218]. In particular, the identification of CR response predictors in patients with schizophrenia is still a topic with equivocal findings and only a few studies have looked for the relationship between CR response or resistance and the biological, sociodemographic, clinical, and cognitive features in schizophrenia [219]. In a recent review of literature, Barlati et al. identify some types of predictors, underlining that CR seems to be more effective in schizophrenia patients with the following features: younger age, shorter duration of illness, few disorganized symptoms, greater pre-treatment cognitive reserve, greater improvement after CR and lower dosages antipsychotics in their current treatment. Regarding CR characteristics, a much larger effect of CR on functioning was found out when a strategic approach was adopted and when CR was offered as part of broader psychosocial rehabilitation interventions. On the other hand, international scientific literature is controversial on the following predictive factors: genetic variability, cognitive and functional impairment at baseline [219]. Moreover, Seccomandi et al. [220] performed a systematic review of the putative factors which may affect CR response, with the aim to identify potential individual factors at baseline, moderators, which may predict treatment outcomes and that may be used to tailor CR and improve its benefits. The authors highlighted five categories of moderators that might influence CR response: demographics, biological, cognitive and functional, psychological, and illness-related characteristics. Nonetheless, they underline that there was no high-quality replicated evidence, which identifies reliable moderators of CR response.

The growing amount of data on CR refers mostly to adult and chronic patients with schizophrenia, but less is known about the effectiveness of CR in the early course of the disease and its possible application on the prodromal phase of the illness [221]. Early phases of the illness are considered a crucial period that could potentially influence its course and during which neural plasticity is thought to play a major pathoplastic role [222–224]. This could justify the theoretical usefulness of interventions targeting cognitive improvement [225]. Revell et al. [226] in their meta-analysis on CR in early schizophrenia underlined that CR in FEP had a positive effect on global cognition; the areas with major results are verbal learning, memory, and social cognition (although only in three of trials). Improvements nearing uncorrected significance were also seen in processing speed, working memory, and in reasoning and problem solving. These results were similar to that reported in the Wykes et al. [19] meta-analysis performed on "chronic" patients, although the ES in FEP review is smaller. The work of Revell et al. [226] reported in conclusion of meta-analytic estimate that CR had a nonsignificant positive effect on global cognition. Nonetheless, this preliminary nonsignificant effect, according to Lewandowski [227], underlines that CR is feasible and potentially efficacious in recent-onset and high-risk patients. This recent review highlights that, in recent-onset patients with schizophrenia, most reports show improvements after CR in one or more domains of cognition. With regard to people at high risk of developing psychosis, some studies report similar promising results although findings on efficacy are inconclusive due to small sample sizes and lack of control [228]. Some studies indicate that effects of CR in these populations may be of similar or greater magnitude as those seen in chronic patients [222], suggesting that young patients with greater potential for plasticity may indeed benefit as much or more than patients with presumably reduced plasticity.

In a recent review, Bellani et al. [229] pay their attention on CR-induced structural and functional brain changes in early SCZ. According to the authors, current literature showed a protective effect of CR on some regions of gray matter volume, as in selected medial temporal (i.e., hippocampus, parahippocampus, and amygdala) and thalamic regions. Functional changes acted on dorsolateral prefrontal and insular cortices both associated with improvements in cognitive performance and emotion regulation. Authors conclude that CR appears to be a promising treatment in the approach to cognitive impairment and neural alterations associated with the early phase of schizophrenia, but future research are needed to clarify whether the positive effects of cognitive training persist over time. In conclusion, preliminary evidence supports the extension of CR in early course and high-risk populations.

2.5.1 Cognitive Remediation: Focus on Psychosocial Functioning

In past decades different outcome measures were recognized as being relevant for effective interventions in schizophrenia such as: quality of life (QoL), obtaining and working competitive jobs, family, and quality of and satisfaction with interpersonal relationships, leisure time, and other elements of daily living, finances, the ability to solve interpersonal problems and physical and mental health [230–232]. Some of these key elements compose psychosocial functioning—defined as patients' ability to fulfil their role in society as a member of a family or in a professional career—that should be a priority target for therapeutic interventions in schizophrenia [233]. As we know starting from scientific literature [8], functional outcome is strongly influenced by cognitive impairment. According to some authors, cognitive deficits explain 20–60% of the variance of real-life functioning [3, 4, 11]. Since these premises, it is crucial that CR could generalize its results and could have an impact on social functioning of patients. Starting from McGurk et al. meta-analysis [196], which includes 26 studies (about 1500 patients), CR programs demonstrate a small/medium ES for functioning (ES, 0.35). Moreover, CR programs that provided adjunctive psychiatric rehabilitation had significantly stronger effects on improving functional outcomes (ES, 0.47) than programs that did not (ES, 0.05). McGurk et al. found that CR intervention, which included strategy coaching, had stronger effects on functioning than programs that focused only on drill and practice techniques. According to the authors, this effect is accordant with previous researches showing that cognitive impairment reduces the response to psychiatric rehabilitation [234–236] and suggests that improved cognitive performance may empower some patients to benefit more from rehabilitation. Also in a previous meta-analysis on CR in schizophrenia, Twamley et al. [192] underlined that all the different types of approaches, whether computer assisted or not, have effective components that are promising for improving everyday functioning. Similar results were found at a later time in Wykes et al. meta-analysis [19], in which CR was associated with a small/medium ES for functioning (ES, 0.35) with a significant heterogeneity in the ES. Stronger ES for improved psychosocial functioning were found by authors in studies that provided adjunctive psychiatric rehabilitation and use of drill and practice plus strategy coaching (ES, 0.62), compared to drill and practice only. This moderator of response could justify the significant heterogeneity in the ES. These findings are also in line with the results of a meta-analysis of integrated psychological therapy—IPT [178], in which the strongest effects on functioning were found in programs that integrated CR and social skills training rather than programs that provided either intervention alone [197, 198].

Furthermore, in 2019 Van Duin et al. performed a meta-analysis in order to investigate whether a combination of psychiatric rehabilitation (PR) and CR reinforces the effect of a stand-alone PR or CR intervention on separate domains of functioning. They analyzed three areas: vocational, social, and community functioning. Regarding vocational functioning, the combination of CR and PR led to significant favorable outcomes for employment rate, hours worked, job duration, and quality of performance in work or education compared with a single PR intervention. Similar results were found in social functioning, in which the combination of CR and PR had significant favorable outcomes for social skills if compared with a single PR intervention. Quite the opposite, no significant beneficial effects were found in community functioning (independent and daily living skills, role adjustment and performance, and social and occupational functioning) when it was compared with a single PR intervention. Results on social and work outcomes were confirmed also by Kambeitz-Ilankovic et al. [205] that found a small, significant effect of CR on functional outcomes. Also the more recent and comprenshive meta-analisys carried-out by Vita et al. [203] underline that the integration of CR into a structured psychiatric rehabilitation program or its association with other evidence-based psychosocial interventions produced better improvements in both cognition and functioning.

With respect to the persistence of the effects on daily functioning, patients treated with the 6 months CRT showed a significant decrease in functional performance after 5 years, compared to the end of treatment. On the contrary, no differences between end of intervention and 5 years later were observed within group that received further standard rehabilitation for a year [201].

Results on functioning were controversial regarding meta-analyses focused only on CACR methods, which seem to be effective in some areas of functioning. On one hand, according to Prikken et al. [204], in patients receiving computerized cognitive drill and practice training compared to a control condition, significant effects on global functional outcomes were absent. On the other, Chan et al. [237], who performed a review on CACR and productivity outcomes, found that CACR can enhance productivity outcomes for patients with severe mental illness (SMI), including higher employment rate, longer duration of work and higher income, improving also quality of life in this population.

Examining results derived from social cognitive training (SCT), we can observe that the first systematic review, which debates this topic [213], concludes that there is also a need for more studies to measure intervention effects on real-world social functioning and that there is potential in including learning strategies (i.e., errorless learning) and harnessing technology (i.e., virtual reality and home-based online training) in order to improve distal outcomes of social competence and social functioning. More promising results derive from the following studies: Grant et al. [212] found a positive effect on functional outcomes used both broad-based and focused studies. The majority of included studies which found an improvement in functioning also reported an improvement in ToM and in social perception. These data support the idea that improvement in ToM may benefit more directly functional outcomes [238], because ToM seems to be relevant in everyday social interactions [239] and because social perception requires the ability to decode social interactions that are strongly associated with functioning improvement. Also, Nijman et al. [217] found that broad-based SCT (with and without CRT) had a significantly larger effect on social functioning, that persists at follow-up. In this meta-analysis, the group treatment was the only variable that significantly moderated the outcome. Concerning CR in in-patients, a recent meta-analysis of Cella et al. [202] showed that there was a positive but no statistically significant effect in favor of CR compared to TAU or TAU plus additional interventions. Authors supposed that assessing social and vocational outcomes in in-patient settings may be difficult because patients may have limited opportunities to practice and take part in activities assessed as part of functional assessment measures.

Significant positive effects of CR were seen on functioning also in FEP [226], with a significantly larger effect in treatments, which employed CR with adjunctive psychiatric rehabilitation (e.g., psychoeducation and training to develop social, vocational, and daily living skills), replicating the findings of the Wykes et al. meta-analysis performed on adult/chronic patients. These results could indicate that targeting cognitive impairments early in the course of the disorder can result not only in cognitive improvement per se, but also in significant functional benefits in such critical domains as employment, social functioning, and major role functioning [221]. In addition, the results could include CR as part of continuing rehabilitation, which may be able to translate cognitive gains directly to better function.

2.5.2 Cognitive Remediation: Focus on Clinical Symptoms

Some small but encouraging results, which infer by CR techniques, were found also in schizophrenia symptoms: as we know from scientific literature, there is a better prognosis in individuals with psychosis, in terms of functioning and symptoms remission, for those with better cognitive performance [240]. Recently it become an established the idea that CR has a direct effect on symptoms. Since the first meta-analytic study was performed on this topic [192], CR (both computer-assisted and not) demonstrated its positive effects on symptoms, with the unknown possibility if these effects were sustainable. Also, two meaningful meta-analytic works agreed with these preliminary results, finding a small significant ES for symptoms [19, 196], that however disappeared at follow-up assessment [19]. A more recent work conducted by Kambeitz-Ilankovic et al. [205], underlines similar effects, finding a small, significant ES of CR on clinical outcomes, particularly in two subdomains: negative and depressive/anxious symptoms. The same results were found in a meta-analysis about CACR training [204], with some small differences: CACR methods showed small/moderate, but only marginally significant effects on negative symptoms and total symptoms, whereas the analysis including all CR methods shows no significant effects on positive, general, and total symptoms, nor on clinical global scores. According to Wykes et al. [19], also Kambeitz-Ilankovic et al. [205] showed no differential response between human guidance of treatment and computerized CR. These results suggest that computerized training programs, which have the potential to be performed independently by patients, are effective [204]. Regarding integrated interventions (for example, IPT), whether they yielded some significant immediate and long-term effects in more proximal outcomes, small effects were found in symptoms [197]. Similar, significant positive effects of CR were seen also in FEP patients on global symptoms: in more detail, CR had a significantly smaller effect on symptoms both when it was delivered one to one with a therapist, as well as when it was delivered in groups [226].

Other specific trainings, for example, social cognitive training programs do not report significant effects on positive and negative symptoms of schizophrenia [195]. According to the authors, the limited effects of social cognitive training on positive and negative symptoms may reflect the multi-determined nature of these disease domains, including emotionally charged family relationships [241]. These interventions produced moderate size effects on general symptoms, suggesting that social cognitive training may be more effective in influencing general psychiatric symptoms such as depression and anxiety.

Furthermore, some studies gave specific attention to CR effect on negative symptoms [242, 243]. Authors underline that negative symptoms are not traditionally considered a primary target for CR, but their results demonstrate a small-to-moderate effect of CR on negative symptoms at post-therapy, with this effect being maintained at follow-up. These findings highlight that CR may have similar ES to other available pharmacological and behavioral interventions designed to tackle negative symptoms directly [244]. Authors suggest that future researches should explore in detail the relationship between cognitive and negative symptoms in schizophrenia. This suggestion was conducted in a recent study exploring the effect of integrated neurocognitive treatment (INT) on relapse rates, which were significantly lower in the INT condition compared with TAU both during therapy and at 1-year follow-up. This analysis points out that the relapse rate after therapy was associated with significant reductions in negative and general symptoms, improvements in functional outcome, and overall cognition. Authors underline that out of these variables, negative symptoms were identified to show the strongest association with relapses after therapy.

2.6 Conclusions and Future Directions

Cognition in schizophrenia is an important target of intervention due to its relationship to outcomes and recovery. In patients with schizophrenia, both social and nonsocial cognitive deficits are related to outcomes and can limit recovery even when another support has been provided [245]. Different pharmacological and non-pharmacological approaches were developed to restore these deficits, although these interventions are still under study and discussed. Some of these treatments, such as SGAs and CR, demonstrate their efficacy also through neuroimaging studies, which underline their neurobiological effects [36, 246]. Furthermore, for each intervention we know that some individuals show little benefit and other much more. This difference leads to an increasing interest in investigating potential moderators, mediators, and predictors of treatment, with the aim to make each treatment tailored for each patient. Despite there are still some future perspectives to observe, different studies support the idea that an integrated approach is required in order to increase everyday functioning and to decrease disability in schizophrenia [168]. To sum up, pharmacological and non-pharmacological approaches moderate both functional improvements and recovery.

References

1. Heinrichs RW, Zakzanis KK. Neurocognitive deficit in schizophrenia: a quantitative review of the evidence. Neuropsychology. 1998;12(3):426–45.
2. Galderisi S, Rossi A, Rocca P, et al. The influence of illness-related variables, personal resources and context-related factors on real-life functioning of people with schizophrenia. World Psychiatry. 2014;13:275–87.
3. Green MF, Kern RS, Heaton RK. Longitudinal studies of cognition and functional outcome in schizophrenia: implications for MATRICS. Schizophr Res. 2004;72:41–51.
4. Green MF, Nuechterlein KH, Gold JM, et al. Approaching a consensus cognitive battery for clinical trials in schizophrenia: the NIMH-MATRICS conference to select cognitive domains and test criteria. Biol Psychiatry. 2004;56(5):301–7.
5. Nuechterlein KH, Green MF, Kern RS, et al. The MATRICS Consensus Cognitive Battery, part 1: test selection, reliability, and validity. Am J Psychiatry. 2008;165(2):203–13.
6. Barch DM, Carter CS, Arnsten A, et al. Selecting paradigms from cognitive neuroscience for translation into use in clinical trials: proceedings of the Third CNTRICS meeting. Schizophr Bull. 2009;35(1):109–14.
7. Couture SM, Penn DL, Roberts DL. The functional significance of social cognition in schizophrenia: a review. Schizophr Bull. 2006;32(1):S44–63.
8. Bowie CR, Reichenberg A, Patterson TL, et al. Determinants of real-world functional performance in schizophrenia subjects: correlations with cognition, functional capacity, and symptoms. Am J Psychiatry. 2006;163(3):418–25.
9. Green MF. What are the functional consequences of neurocognitive deficits in schizophrenia? Am J Psychiatry. 1996;153(3):321–30.
10. Green MF, Kern RS, Braff DL, et al. Neurocognitive deficits and functional outcome in schizophrenia: are we measuring the "right stuff"? Schizophr Bull. 2000;26(1):119–36.

11. Fett AK, Viechtbauer W, Dominguez MD, et al. The relationship between neurocognition and social cognition with functional outcomes in schizophrenia: a meta-analysis. Neurosci Biobehav Rev. 2016;35:573–88.
12. Green MF, Nuechterlein KH, Kern RS, et al. Functional co-primary measures for clinical trials in schizophrenia: results from the MATRICS Psychometric and Standardization Study. Am J Psychiatry. 2008;165(2):221–8.
13. Bowie CR, Leung WW, Reichenberg A, et al. Predicting schizophrenia patients' real-world behavior with specific neuropsychological and functional capacity measures. Biol Psychiatry. 2008;63(5):505–11.
14. Galderisi S, Rossi A, Rocca P, et al. Pathways to functional outcome in subjects with schizophrenia living in the community and their unaffected first-degree relatives. Schizophr Res. 2016;175:154–60.
15. Medalia A, Choi J. Cognitive remediation in schizophrenia. Neuropsychol Rev. 2009;19:353–64.
16. Martin DM, McClintock SM, Forster J, et al. Does therapeutic repetitive transcranial magnetic stimulation cause cognitive enhancing effects in patients with neuropsychiatric conditions? A systematic review and meta-analysis of randomised controlled trials. Neuropsychol Rev. 2016;26(3):295–309.
17. Maurus I, Röh A, Falkai P, Malchow B, Schmitt A, Hasan A. Nonpharmacological treatment of dyscognition in schizophrenia: effects of aerobic exercise. Dialogues Clin Neurosci. 2019;21(3):261–9.
18. McCleery A, Nuechterlein KH. Cognitive impairment in psychotic illness: prevalence, profile of impairment, developmental course, and treatment considerations. Dialogues Clin Neurosci. 2019;21(3):239–48.
19. Wykes T, Huddy V, et al. A meta-analysis of cognitive remediation of schizophrenia: methodology and effect sizes. Am J Psychiatry. 2011;168:472–85.
20. Yu L, Fang X, Chen Y, et al. Efficacy of transcranial direct current stimulation in ameliorating negative symptoms and cognitive impairments in schizophrenia: a systematic review and meta-analysis. Schizophr Res. 2020;224:2–10.
21. Keshavan M, Eack S. Psychopharmacological approaches, cognitive enhancement, and brain stimulation. In: Cognitive enhancement in schizophrenia and related disorders. Cambridge: Cambridge University Press; 2019. p. 90–102.
22. Mackenzie NE, Kowalchuk C, et al. Antipsychotics, metabolic adverse effects, and cognitive function in schizophrenia. Front Psychiatry. 2018;9:622.
23. Bora E, Akdede BB, Alptekin K. Neurocognitive impairment in deficit and non-deficit schizophrenia: a meta-analysis. Psychol Med. 2017;47(14):2401–13.
24. Botis AC, Miclutia I, Vlasin N. Cognitive function in female patients with schizophrenia and metabolic syndrome. Eur Psychiatry. 2016;33:97.
25. Boyer L, Richieri R, Dassa D, et al. Association of metabolic syndrome and inflammation with neurocognition in patients with schizophrenia. Psychiatry Res. 2013;210(2):381–6.
26. Lindenmayer JP, Khan A, Kaushik S. Relationship between metabolic syndrome and cognition in patients with schizophrenia. Schizophr Res. 2012;142(1–3):171–6.
27. Bora E, Akdede BB, Alptekin K. The relationship between cognitive impairment in schizophrenia and metabolic syndrome: a systematic review and meta-analysis. Psychol Med. 2017;47(6):1030–40.
28. Storch-Jakobsen A, Speyer H, et al. Associations between clinical and psychosocial factors and metabolic and cardiovascular risk factors in overweight patients with schizophrenia spectrum disorders - baseline and two-years findings from the CHANGE trial. Schizophr Res. 2018;199:96–102.
29. Friedman JI, Wallenstein S, Moshier E, et al. The effects of hypertension and body mass index on cognition in schizophrenia. Am J Psychiatry. 2010;167(10):1232–9.
30. Goughari AS, Mazhari S, Pourrahimi AM, et al. Associations between components of metabolic syndrome and cognition in patients with schizophrenia. J Psychiatr Pract. 2015;21(3):190–7.

31. Mitchell AJ, Vancampfort D, Sweers K. Prevalence of metabolic syndrome and metabolic abnormalities in schizophrenia and related disorders—a systematic review and meta-analysis. Schizophr Bull. 2013;39(2):306–18.
32. Lieberman JA. Is schizophrenia a neurodegenerative disorder? A clinical and neurobiological perspective. Biol Psychiatry. 1999;46:729–39.
33. Nikam SS, Awasthi AK. Evolution of schizophrenia drugs: a focus on dopaminergic systems. Curr Opin Investig Drugs. 2008;9:37–46.
34. Veselinović T, Scharpenberg M, et al. Disparate effects of first- and second-generation antipsychotics on cognition in schizophrenia – findings from the randomized NeSSy trial. Eur Neuropsychopharmacol. 2019;29:720–39.
35. Gallhofer B, Bauer U, Lis S, et al. Cognitive dysfunction in schizophrenia: comparison of treatment with atypical antipsychotic agents and conventional neuroleptic drugs. Eur Neuropsychopharmacol. 1996;6(2):S13–20.
36. Vita A, De Peri L, Deste G, Barlati S, Sacchetti E. The effect of antipsychotic treatment on cortical gray matter changes in schizophrenia: does the class matter? A meta-analysis and meta-regression of longitudinal magnetic resonance imaging studies. Biol Psychiatry. 2015;78(6):403–12.
37. Meltzer HY, Huang M. In vivo actions of atypical antipsychotic drug on serotonergic and dopaminergic systems. Prog Brain Res. 2008;172:177–97.
38. Ichikawa J, Dai J, O'Laughlin IA, et al. Atypical, but not typical, antipsychotic drugs increase cortical acetylcholine release without an effect in the nucleus accumbens or striatum. Neuropsychopharmacology. 2002;26:325–39.
39. Torrisi SA, Laudani S, Contarini G, et al. Dopamine, cognitive impairments and second-generation antipsychotics: from mechanistic advances to more personalized treatments. Pharmaceuticals. 2020;13(11):365.
40. Meltzer HY. The role of serotonin in antipsychotic drug action. Neuropsychopharmacology. 1999;21:106S–15S.
41. Ichikawa J, Ishii H, Bonaccorso S, et al. 5-HT(2A) and D(2) receptor blockade increases cortical DA release via 5-HT(1A) receptor activation: a possible mechanism of atypical antipsychotic-induced cortical dopamine release. J Neurochem. 2001;76:1521–31.
42. Bymaster FP, Felder CC, Tzavara E, et al. Muscarinic mechanisms of antipsychotic atypicality. Prog Neuropsychopharmacol Biol Psychiatry. 2003;27:1125–43.
43. Carpenter WT, Gold JM. Another view of therapy for cognition in schizophrenia. Biol Psychiatry. 2002;51:969–71.
44. Correll CU, Lencz T, Malhotra AK. Antipsychotic drugs and obesity. Trends Mol Med. 2011;17(2):97–107.
45. Davidson M, Galderisi S, Weiser M, et al. Cognitive effects of antipsychotic drugs in first-episode schizophrenia and schizophreniform disorder: a randomized, open-label clinical trial (EUFEST). Am J Psychiatry. 2009;166:675–82.
46. Mortimer AM, Joyce E, Balasubramaniam K, et al. SOLIANOL Study Group. Treatment with amisulpride and olanzapine improve neuropsychological function in schizophrenia. Hum Psychopharmacol. 2007;22:445–54.
47. Bervoets C, Morrens M, Vansteelandt K, et al. Effect of aripiprazole on verbal memory and fluency in schizophrenic patients: results from the ESCAPE study. CNS Drugs. 2012;26:975–82.
48. Gooze R, Reinders AA, Handley R, et al. Effects of aripiprazole and haloperidol on neural activation during the n-back in healthy individuals: a functional MRI study. Schizophr Res. 2016;173:174–81.
49. Potkin S, Fleming K, Binnerman B, et al. Effects of asenapine on cognitive function in acute schizophrenia: a placebo- and risperidone-controlled trial. Eur Neuropsychopharmacol. 2007;17:S466–7.
50. Corponi F, Fabbri C, Bitter I, et al. Novel antipsychotics specificity profile: a clinically oriented review of lurasidone, brexpiprazole, cariprazine and lumateperone. Eur Neuropsychopharmacol. 2019;29(9):971–85.

51. Fleischhacker WW, Hobart M, Ouyang J, et al. Efficacy and safety of brexpiprazole (OPC-34712) as maintenance treatment in adults with schizophrenia: a randomized, double-blind, placebo-controlled study. Int J Neuropsychopharmacol. 2017;20:11–21.
52. Neill JC, Grayson B, Kiss B, et al. Effects of cariprazine, a novel antipsychotic, on cognitive deficit and negative symptoms in a rodent model of schizophrenia symptomatology. Eur Neuropsychopharmacol. 2016;26:3–14.
53. Werner FM, Coveñas R. The novel antipsychotic drug cariprazine and cognition enhancing drugs: indications for their use as an add-on therapy in schizophrenia. Curr Pharm Des. 2021;27(39):4033–8.
54. Meltzer HY, McGurk SR. The effects of clozapine, risperidone, and olanzapine on cognitive function in schizophrenia. Schizophr Bull. 1999;25:233–55.
55. Woodward ND, Purdon SE, Meltzer HY, et al. A meta-analysis of neuropsychological change to clozapine, olanzapine, quetiapine, and risperidone in schizophrenia. Int J Neuropsychopharmacol. 2005;8:457–72.
56. Ishibashi T, Horisawa T, Tokuda K, et al. Pharmacological profile of lurasidone, a novel antipsychotic agent with potent 5-hydroxytryptamine 7 (5-HT7) and 5-HT1A receptor activity. J Pharmacol Exp Ther. 2010;334(1):171–81.
57. Harvey PD, Siu CO, Ogasa M, et al. Effect of lurasidone dose on cognition in patients with schizophrenia: post-hoc analysis of a long-term, double-blind continuation study. Schizophr Res. 2015;166(1–3):334–8.
58. Kim SW, Chung YC, Lee YH, et al. Paliperidone ER versus risperidone for neuro cognitive function in patients with schizophrenia: a randomized, open-label, controlled trial. Int Clin Psychopharmacol. 2012;27:267–74.
59. Johnsen E, Jørgensen HA, Kroken RA, et al. Neurocognitive effectiveness of quetiapine, olanzapine, risperidone, and ziprasidone: a pragmatic, randomized trial. Eur Psychiatry. 2013;28(3):174–84.
60. McGurk SR, Lee MA, Jayathilake K, et al. Cognitive effects of olanzapine treatment in schizophrenia. Med Gen Med. 2004;6:27.
61. Wang CH, Li Y, Yang J, et al. A randomized controlled trial of olanzapine improving memory deficits in Han Chinese patients with first-episode schizophrenia. Schizophr Res. 2013;144:129–35.
62. Kern RS, Green MF, Cornblatt BA. The neurocognitive effects of aripiprazole: an open-label comparison with olanzapine. Psychopharmacology. 2006;187:312–20.
63. Houthoofd SA, Morrens M, Sabbe BG. Cognitive and psychomotor effects of risperidone in schizophrenia and schizoaffective disorder. Clin Ther. 2008;30:1565–89.
64. Maat A, Cahn W, Gijsman HJ, et al. Open, randomized trial of the effects of aripiprazole versus risperidone on social cognition in schizophrenia. Eur Neuropsychopharmacol. 2014;24:575–84.
65. Park JH, Hong JS, Kim SM, et al. Effects of amisulpride adjunctive therapy on working memory and brain metabolism in the frontal cortex of patients with schizophrenia: a preliminary positron emission tomography/computerized tomography investigation. Clin Psychopharmacol Neurosci. 2019;17(2):250–60.
66. Nielsen RE, Levander S, Kjaersdam Telleus G, et al. Second-generation antipsychotic effect on cognition in patients with schizophrenia—a meta-analysis of randomized clinical trials. Acta Psychiatr Scand. 2015;131:185–96.
67. Clissold M, Crowe SF. Comparing the effect of the subcategories of atypical antipsychotic medications on cognition in schizophrenia using a meta-analytic approach. J Clin Exp Neuropsychol. 2019;41(1):26–42.
68. Désaméricq G, Schurhoff F, Meary A, et al. Long-term neurocognitive effects of antipsychotics in schizophrenia: a network meta-analysis. Eur J Clin Pharmacol. 2014;70(2):127–34.
69. Kahn RS, Sommer IE. The neurobiology and treatment of first-episode schizophrenia. Mol Psychiatry. 2015;20(1):84–97.

70. Hori H, Katsuki A, Atake K, et al. Effects of continuing oral risperidone vs. switching from risperidone to risperidone long-acting injection on cognitive function in stable schizophrenia patients: a pilot study. Front Psychiatry. 2018;9:74.
71. Takekita Y, Koshikawa Y, Fabbri C, et al. Cognitive function and risperidone long-acting injection vs paliperidone palmitate in schizophrenia: a 6-month, open-label, randomized, pilot trial. BMC Psychiatry. 2016;16:172.
72. Leucht S, Corves C, Arbter D, et al. Second generation versus first-generation antipsychotic drugs for schizophrenia: a meta-analysis. Lancet. 2009;373(9657):31–41.
73. Leucht S, Komossa K, Rummel-Kluge C, et al. A meta-analysis of head-to-head comparisons of second-generation antipsychotics in the treatment of schizophrenia. Am J Psychiatry. 2009;166:152–63.
74. McEvoy JP. A double-blind crossover comparison of antiparkinson drug therapy: amantadine versus anticholinergics in 90 normal volunteers, with an emphasis on differential effects on memory function. J Clin Psychiatry. 1987;48:S20–3.
75. Spohn HE, Strauss ME. Relation of neuroleptic and anticholinergic medication to cognitive functions in schizophrenia. J Abnorm Psychol. 1989;98:367–80.
76. Guillena SLR, Garcia de Dego BOP. Cognitive impairment in schizophrenia. First-generation long-acting antipsychotics versus aripiprazole long-acting injectable. Cambridge: Cambridge University Press; 2019. p. 211–2.
77. Han L, McCusker J, Cole M, et al. Antidepressant use and cognitive functioning in older medical patients with major or minor depression: a prospective cohort study with database linkage. J Clin Psychopharmacol. 2011;31:429–35.
78. Herrera-Guzman I, Gudayol-Ferre E, et al. Major depressive disorder in recovery and neuropsychological functioning: effects of selective serotonin reuptake inhibitor and dual inhibitor depression treatments on residual cognitive deficits in patients with major depressive disorder in recovery. J Affect Disord. 2010;123:341–50.
79. McIntyre RS, Lophaven S, Olsen CK. A randomized, double-blind, placebo-controlled study of vortioxetine on cognitive function in depressed adults. Int J Neuropsychopharmacol. 2014;17:1557–67.
80. Pehrson AL, Sanchez C. Serotonergic modulation of glutamate neurotransmission as a strategy for treating depression and cognitive dysfunction. CNS Spectr. 2014;19:121–33.
81. Friedman JI, Ocampo R, Elbaz Z, et al. The effect of citalopram adjunctive treatment added to atypical antipsychotic medications for cognitive performance in patients with schizophrenia. J Clin Psychopharmacol. 2005;25:237–42.
82. Evins AE, Deckersbach T, Cather C. Independent effects of tobacco abstinence and bupropion on cognitive function in schizophrenia. J Clin Psychiatry. 2005;66:1184–90.
83. Stenberg JH, Terevnikov V, Joffe M, et al. Effects of add-on mirtazapine on neurocognition in schizophrenia: a double-blind, randomized, placebo-controlled study. Int J Neuropsychopharmacol. 2010;13:433–41.
84. Poyurovsky M, Koren D, Gonopolsky I, et al. Effect of the 5-HT2 antagonist mianserin on cognitive dysfunction in chronic schizophrenia patients: an add-on, double-blind placebo-controlled study. Eur Neuropsychopharmacol. 2003;13:123–8.
85. Vernon JA, Grudnikoff E, Seidman AJ, et al. Antidepressants for cognitive impairment in schizophrenia-a systematic review and meta-analysis. Schizophr Res. 2014;159(2–3):385–94.
86. Hecht EM, Landy DC. Alpha-2 receptor antagonist add-on therapy in the treatment of schizophrenia: a meta-analysis. Schizophr Res. 2012;134(2–3):202–6.
87. Moazen-Zadeh E, Bayanati S, Ziafat K, et al. Vortioxetine as adjunctive therapy to risperidone for treatment of patients with chronic schizophrenia: a randomised, double-blind, placebo-controlled clinical trial. J Psychopharmacol. 2020;34(5):506–13.
88. Rummel C, Kissling W, Leucht S. Antidepressants for the negative symptoms of schizophrenia. Cochrane Database Syst Rev. 2006;3:CD005581.
89. Sepehry AA, Potvin S, Elie R, et al. Selective serotonin reuptake inhibitor (SSRI) add-on therapy for the negative symptoms of schizophrenia: a meta-analysis. J Clin Psychiatry. 2007;68:604–10.

90. Singh SP, Singh V, Kar N, et al. Efficacy of antidepressants in treating the negative symptoms of chronic schizophrenia: meta-analysis. Br J Psychiatry. 2010;197:174–9.
91. Whitehead C, Moss S, Cardno A, et al. Antidepressants for the treatment of depression in people with schizophrenia: a systematic review. Psychol Med. 2003;33:589–99.
92. Miyamoto S, Miyake N, Jarskog LF, et al. Pharmacological treatment of schizophrenia: a critical review of the pharmacology and clinical effects of current and future therapeutic agents. Mol Psychiatry. 2012;17(12):1206–27.
93. Jones P, Rodgers B, Murray R, et al. Child development risk factors for adult schizophrenia in the British 1946 Birth Cohort. Lancet. 1994;344(8934):1398–402.
94. Beasley CL, Zhang ZJ, Patten I, et al. Selective deficits in prefrontal cortical GABAergic neurons in schizophrenia defined by the presence of calcium-binding proteins. Biol Psychiatry. 2002;52:708–15.
95. Kegeles LS, Mao X, Stanford AD, et al. Elevated prefrontal cortex gamma-aminobutyric acid and glutamate-glutamine levels in schizophrenia measured in vivo with proton magnetic resonance spectroscopy. Arch Gen Psychiatry. 2012;69:449–59.
96. Olney JW, Newcomer JW, Farber NB. NMDA receptor hypofunction model of schizophrenia. J Psychiatr Res. 1999;33:523–33.
97. Genius J, Giegling I, Benninghoff J, et al. Disturbed function of GABAergic interneurons in schizophrenia: relevance for medical treatment? Curr Pharm Biotechnol. 2012;13:1549–56.
98. Lewis DA, Volk DW, Hashimoto T. Selective alterations in prefrontal cortical GABA neurotransmission in schizophrenia: a novel target for the treatment of working memory dysfunction. Psychopharmacology. 2004;174:143–50.
99. Harvey PD. Pharmacological cognitive enhancement in schizophrenia. Neuropsychol Rev. 2009;19:324–35.
100. Uehara T, Sumiyoshi T, Kurachi M. New pharmacotherapy targeting cognitive dysfunction of schizophrenia via modulation of GABA neuronal function. Curr Neuropharmacol. 2015;13:793–801.
101. Lewis DA, Cho RY, Carter CS, et al. Subunit-selective modulation of GABA type A receptor neurotransmission and cognition in schizophrenia. Am J Psychiatry. 2008;165:1585–93.
102. Moghaddam B, Javitt D. From revolution to evolution: the glutamate hypothesis of schizophrenia and its implication for treatment. Neuropsychopharmacology. 2012;37:4–15.
103. Heresco-Levy U, Javitt DC, et al. Double-blind, placebo-controlled crossover trial of glycine adjuvant therapy for treatment-resistant schizophrenia. Br J Psychiatry. 1996;169:610–7.
104. Lucas-Meunier E, Fossier P, Baux G, et al. Cholinergic modulation of the cortical neuronal network. Pflugers Arch. 2003;446:17–29.
105. Tandon R. Antipsychotics in the treatment of schizophrenia: an overview. J Clin Psychiatry. 2011;72(1):4–8.
106. Thomas E, Snyder PJ, Pietrzak RH, et al. Specific impairments in visuospatial working and short-term memory following low-dose scopolamine challenge in healthy older adults. Neuropsychologia. 2008;46:2476–84.
107. Gibbons AS, Scarr E, Boer S, et al. Widespread decreases in cortical muscarinic receptors in a subset of people with schizophrenia. Int J Neuropsychopharmacol. 2013;16:37–46.
108. Zavitsanou K, Garrick T, Huang XF. Selective antagonist [3H]SR141716A binding to cannabinoid CB1 receptors is increased in the anterior cingulate cortex in schizophrenia. Prog Neuropsychopharmacol Biol Psychiatry. 2004;28:355–60.
109. Carruthers SP, Gurvich CT, Rossell SL. The muscarinic system, cognition and schizophrenia. Neurosci Biobehav Rev. 2015;55:393–402.
110. Bilder RM, Goldman RS, Volavka J, et al. Neurocognitive effects of clozapine, olanzapine, risperidone, and haloperidol in patients with chronic schizophrenia or schizoaffective disorder. Am J Psychiatry. 2002;159:1018–28.
111. Lilienfeld S. Galantamine—a novel cholinergic drug with a unique dual mode of action for the treatment of patients with Alzheimer's disease. CNS Drug Rev. 2002;8:159–76.

112. Buchanan RW, Conley RR, Dickinson D, et al. Galantamine for the treatment of cognitive impairments in people with schizophrenia. Am J Psychiatry. 2008;165:82–9.
113. Deutsch SI, Schwartz BL, Schooler NR, et al. Targeting alpha-7 nicotinic neurotransmission in schizophrenia: a novel agonist strategy. Schizophr Res. 2013;148:138–44.
114. Nickols HH, Conn PJ. Development of allosteric modulators of GPCRs for treatment of CNS disorders. Neurobiol Dis. 2014;61:55–71.
115. Chambon C, Jatzke C, Wegener N, et al. Using cholinergic M1 receptor positive allosteric modulators to improve memory via enhancement of brain cholinergic communication. Eur J Pharmacol. 2012;697:73–80.
116. Vardigan JD, Cannon CE, Puri V, et al. Improved cognition without adverse effects: novel M1 muscarinic potentiator compares favorably to donepezil and xanomeline in rhesus monkey. Psychopharmacology. 2015;232:1859–66.
117. Bubser M, Bridges TM, Dencker D, et al. Selective activation of M4 muscarinic acetylcholine receptors reverses MK-801-induced behavioral impairments and enhances associative learning in rodents. ACS Chem Neurosci. 2014;5:920–42.
118. Galloway CR, Lebois EP, Shagarabi SL, et al. Effects of selective activation of m1 and m4 muscarinic receptors on object recognition memory performance in rats. Pharmacology. 2014;93:57–64.
119. Koukouli F, Changeux JP. Do nicotinic receptors modulate high-order cognitive processing? Trends Neurosci. 2020;43(8):550–64.
120. Huang M, Felix AR, Flood DG, et al. The novel α7 nicotinic acetylcholine receptor agonist EVP-6124 enhances dopamine, acetylcholine, and glutamate efflux in rat cortex and nucleus accumbens. Psychopharmacology. 2014;231:4541–51.
121. Keefe RSE, Meltzer HA, Dgetluck N, et al. Randomized, double-blind, placebo-controlled study of encenicline, an α7 nicotinic acetylcholine receptor agonist, as a treatment for cognitive impairment in schizophrenia. Neuropsychopharmacology. 2015;40:3053–60.
122. Kas MJ, Penninx B, Sommer B, et al. A quantitative approach to neuropsychiatry: the why and the how. Neurosci Biobehav Rev. 2019;97:3–9.
123. Chung Y-C, Lee C-R, Park T-W, et al. Effect of donepezil added to atypical antipsychotics on cognition in patients with schizophrenia: an open-label trial. World J Biol Psychiatry. 2009;10:156–62.
124. Choi KH, Wykes T, Kurtz MM. Adjunctive pharmacotherapy for cognitive deficits in schizophrenia: meta-analytical investigation of efficacy. Br J Psychiatry. 2013;203:172–8.
125. Swerdlow NR, Bhakta S, Chou HH, et al. Memantine effects on sensorimotor gating and mismatch negativity in patients with chronic psychosis. Neuropsychopharmacology. 2016;41:419–30.
126. Lieberman JA, Drake RE, Sederer LI, et al. Science and recovery in schizophrenia. Psychiatr Serv. 2008;59(5):487–96.
127. Lieberman JA, Papadakis K, Csernansky J, et al. A randomized, placebo-controlled study of memantine as adjunctive treatment in patients with schizophrenia. Neuropsychopharmacology. 2008;34:1322–9.
128. Bukovskaya O, Shmukler A. Oxytocin and social cognitions in schizophrenia: a systematic review. Psychiatry Q. 2016;87(3):521–43.
129. Friedman JI, Adler DN, Temporini HD, et al. Guanfacine treatment of cognitive impairment in schizophrenia. Neuropsychopharmacology. 2001;25:402–9.
130. Friedman JI, Carpenter D, Lu J, et al. A pilot study of adjunctive atomoxetine treatment to second generation antipsychotics for cognitive impairment in schizophrenia. J Clin Psychopharmacol. 2008;28:59–63.
131. Poyurovsky M, Faragian S, Fuchs C, et al. Effect of the selective norepinephrine reuptake inhibitor reboxetine on cognitive dysfunction in schizophrenia patients: an addon, double-blind placebo-controlled study. Isr J Psychiatry Relat Sci. 2009;46:213–20.
132. Sumiyoshi T, Matsui M, Nohara S, et al. Enhancement of cognitive performance in schizophrenia by addition of tandospirone to neuroleptic treatment. Am J Psychiatry. 2001;158(10):1722–5.

133. Piskulić D, Olver JS, Maruff P, et al. Treatment of cognitive dysfunction in chronic schizophrenia by augmentation of atypical antipsychotics with buspirone, a partial 5-HT(1A) receptor agonist. Hum Psychopharmacol. 2009;24:437–46.
134. Zhang Z-J, Kang W-H, Li Q, et al. Beneficial effects of ondansetron as an adjunct to haloperidol for chronic, treatment-resistant schizophrenia: a double-blind, randomized, placebo-controlled study. Schizophr Res. 2006;88:102–10.
135. Meyer U, Feldon J, Yee BK. A review of the fetal brain cytokine imbalance hypothesis of schizophrenia. Schizophr Bull. 2009;35:959–72.
136. Forrest CM, Khalil OS, Pisar M, et al. Prenatal activation of Toll-like receptors-3 by administration of the viral mimetic poly(I:C) changes synaptic proteins, N-methyl-D-aspartate receptors and neurogenesis markers in offspring. Mol Brain. 2012;5:22.
137. Miller BJ, Buckley P, Seabolt W, et al. Metaanalysis of cytokine alterations in schizophrenia: clinical status and antipsychotic effects. Biol Psychiatry. 2011;70:663–71.
138. Campbell IL, Abraham CR, Masliah E, et al. Neurologic disease induced in transgenic mice by cerebral overexpression of interleukin 6. PNAS. 1993;90:10061–5.
139. Sullivan EM, O'Donnell P. Inhibitory interneurons, oxidative stress, and schizophrenia. Schizophr Bull. 2012;38:373–6.
140. Dickerson F, Stallings C, Origoni A, et al. C-reactive protein is associated with the severity of cognitive impairment but not of psychiatric symptoms in individuals with schizophrenia. Schizophr Res. 2007;93:261–5.
141. Karanikas EP. Psycho-immunological mechanisms in schizophrenia. Psychiatrike. 2011;22:43–52.
142. Çakici N, van Beveren NJM, Judge-Hundal G, et al. An update on the efficacy of anti-inflammatory agents for patients with schizophrenia: a meta-analysis. Psychol Med. 2019;49(14):2307–19.
143. Sironi L, Gianazza E, Gelosa P, et al. Rosuvastatin, but not simvastatin, provides end-organ protection in stroke-prone rats by anti-inflammatory effects. Arterioscler Thromb Vasc Biol. 2005;25:598–603.
144. Minzenberg MJ, Carter CS. Modafinil: a review of neurochemical actions and effects on cognition. Neuropsychopharmacology. 2008;33:1477–502.
145. Ishizuka T, Murakami M, Yamatodani A. Involvement of central histaminergic systems in modafinil-induced but not methylphenidate-induced increases in locomotor activity in rats. Eur J Pharmacol. 2008;578:209–15.
146. Lees J, Michalopoulou PG, Lewis SW, et al. Modafinil and cognitive enhancement in schizophrenia and healthy volunteers: the effects of test battery in a randomised controlled trial. Psychol Med. 2017;47(13):2358–68.
147. Andrade C, Kisely S, Monteiro I, et al. Antipsychotic augmentation with modafinil or armodafinil for negative symptoms of schizophrenia: systematic review and meta-analysis of randomized controlled trials. J Psychiatr Res. 2015;60:14–21.
148. Ortiz-Orendain J, Covarrubias-Castillo SA, Vazquez-Alvarez AO, et al. Modafinil for people with schizophrenia or related disorders. Cochrane Database Syst Rev. 2019;12(12):CD008661.
149. McNamara RK, Carlson SE. Role of omega-3 fatty acids in brain development and function: potential implications for the pathogenesis and prevention of psychopathology. Prostaglandins Leukot Essent Fatty Acids. 2006;75:329–49.
150. Amminger GP, Schafer MR, Klier CM, et al. Decreased nervonic acid levels in erythrocyte membranes predict psychosis in help-seeking ultra-high-risk individuals. Mol Psychiatry. 2012;17:1150–2.
151. Farokhnia M, Azarkolah A, Adinehfar F, et al. N-acetylcysteine as an adjunct to risperidone for treatment of negative symptoms in patients with chronic schizophrenia: a randomized, doubleblind, placebo-controlled study. Clin Neuropharmacol. 2013;36:185–92.
152. Bossong MG, Jansma JM, Bhattacharyya S. Role of the endocannabinoid system in brain functions relevant for schizophrenia: an overview of human challenge studies with cannabis or Δ9-tetrahydrocannabinol (THC). Prog Neuropsychopharmacol Biol Psychiatry. 2014;52:53–69.

153. Zavitsanou K, Katerina Z, Katsifis A, et al. Investigation of m1/m4 muscarinic receptors in the anterior cingulate cortex in schizophrenia, bipolar disorder, and major depression disorder. Neuropsychopharmacology. 2004;29:619–25.
154. Burstein S. Cannabidiol (CBD) and its analogs: a review of their effects on inflammation. Bioorg Med Chem. 2015;23:1377–85.
155. Hahn B. The potential of cannabidiol treatment for cannabis users with recent-onset psychosis. Schizophr Bull. 2018;44(1):46–53.
156. Kopelli E, Samara M, Siargkas A, et al. The role of cannabidiol oil in schizophrenia treatment. A systematic review and meta-analysis. Psychiatry Res. 2020;291:113246.
157. Osborne AL, Solowij N, Weston-Green K. A systematic review of the effect of cannabidiol on cognitive function: relevance to schizophrenia. Neurosci Biobehav Rev. 2017;72:310–24.
158. Chang CH, Lane HY, Tseng PT, et al. Effect of N-methyl-D-aspartate-receptor-enhancing agents on cognition in patients with schizophrenia: a systematic review and meta-analysis of double-blind randomised controlled trials. J Psychopharmacol. 2019;33(4):436–48.
159. Robbins TW. Pharmacological treatment of cognitive deficits in nondementing mental health disorders. Dialogues Clin Neurosci. 2019;21(3):301–8.
160. Talpos JC. Symptomatic thinking: the current state of phase III and IV clinical trials for cognition in schizophrenia. Drug Discov Today. 2017;22(7):1017–26.
161. Yang YS, Marder SR, Green MF. Repurposing drugs for cognition in schizophrenia. Clin Pharmacol Ther. 2017;101(2):191–3.
162. Jones C. α7 nicotinic acetylcholine receptor: a potential target in treating cognitive decline in schizophrenia. J Clin Psychopharmacol. 2018;38(3):247–9.
163. Takano H. Cognitive function and monoamine neurotransmission in schizophrenia: evidence from positron emission tomography studies. Front Psych. 2018;29(9):228.
164. Zheng W, Cai DB, Zhang QE, et al. Adjunctive ondansetron for schizophrenia: a systematic review and meta-analysis of randomized controlled trials. J Psychiatr Res. 2019 Jun;113:27–33.
165. Koola MM. Antipsychotic-minocycline-acetylcysteine combination for positive, cognitive, and negative symptoms of schizophrenia. Asian J Psychiatr. 2019;40:100–2.
166. Knöchel C, Voss M, Grüter F, et al. Omega 3 fatty acids: novel neurotherapeutic targets for cognitive dysfunction in mood disorders and schizophrenia? Curr Neuropharmacol. 2015;13(5):663–80.
167. Rapado-Castro M, Dodd S, Bush AI, et al. Cognitive effects of adjunctive N-acetyl cysteine in psychosis. Psychol Med. 2017;47(5):866–76.
168. Vita A, Barlati S. Recovery from schizophrenia: is it possible? Curr Opin Psychiatry. 2018;31(3):246–55.
169. Kaneko Y, Keshavan M. Cognitive remediation in schizophrenia. Clin Psychopharmacol Neurosci. 2012;10:125–35.
170. Eack SM, Hogarty GE, Cho RY, et al. Neuroprotective effects of cognitive enhancement therapy against gray matter loss in early schizophrenia: results from a 2-year randomized controlled trial. Arch Gen Psychiatry. 2010;67(7):674–82.
171. Bowie CR, McGurk SR, Mausbach B, et al. Combined cognitive remediation and functional skills training for schizophrenia: effects on cognition, functional competence, and real-world behavior. Am J Psychiatry. 2012;169(7):710–8.
172. Sohlberg MM, Mateer CA. Training use of compensatory memory books: a three stage behavioral approach. J Clin Exp Neuropsychol. 1989;11(6):871–91.
173. Vita A, Barlati S, Bellani M, et al. Cognitive remediation in schizophrenia: background, techniques, evidence of efficacy and perspectives. Epidemiol Psychiatr Sci. 2014;23(1):21–5.
174. Best MW, Bowie CR. A review of cognitive remediation approaches for schizophrenia: from top-down to bottom-up, brain training to psychotherapy. Expert Rev Neurother. 2017;17(7):713–23.
175. Medalia A, Lim R. Treatment of cognitive dysfunction in psychiatric disorders. J Psychiatr Pract. 2004;10(1):17–25.
176. Wykes T, Reeder C. Cognitive remediation therapy for schizophrenia. Theory and practice. London: Routledge; 1999.

177. Cella M, Reeder C, Wykes T. Cognitive remediation in schizophrenia—now it is really getting personal. Curr Opin Behav Sci. 2015;4:147–51.
178. Brenner H, Roder V, Hodel B, et al. Integrated psychological therapy for schizophrenic patients. Seattle: Hogrefe & Huber; 1994.
179. Bell M, Bryson G, Greig T, et al. Neurocognitive enhancement therapy with work therapy: effects on neuropsychological test performance. Arch Gen Psychiatry. 2001;58(8):763–8.
180. Medalia A, Revheim N, Casey M. Remediation of problem-solving skills in schizophrenia: evidence of a persistent effect. Schizophr Res. 2002;57(2–3):165–71.
181. Hogarty GE, Greenwald DP. Cognitive Enhancement Therapy: The Training Manual. University of Pittsburgh Medical Center, 2006.
182. Roder V, Mueller DR. Integrated Neurocognitive Therapy (INT) for Schizophrenia Patients. University Psychiatric Hospital, Bern, Switzerland, 2006.
183. Galderisi S, Piegari G, Mucci A et al. Social skills and neurocognitive individualized training in schizophrenia: comparison with structured leisure activities. Eur Arch Psychiatry Clin Neurosci. 2010;260(4):305–15.
184. Wölwer W, Frommann N, Halfmann S, et al. Remediation of impairments in facial affect recognition in schizophrenia: efficacy and specificity of a new training program. Schizophr Res. 2005;80(2–3):295–303.
185. Penn D, Roberts DL, Munt ED, et al. A pilot study of social cognition and interaction training (SCIT) for schizophrenia. Schizophr Res. 2005;80(2–3):357–59.
186. Choi K, Kwon J. Social cognition enhancement training for schizophrenia: a preliminary randomized controlled trial. Community Ment Health J. 2006;42(2):177–87.
187. Horan WP, Kern RS, Tripp C et al. Efficacy and specificity of Social Cognitive Skills Training for outpatients with psychotic disorders. J Psychiatr Res. 2011;45(8):1113–22.
188. Reeder C, Wykes T. Computerised interactive remediation of cognition—interactive training for schizophrenia (CIRCUITS). London: Kings College London; 2010.
189. Twamley EW, Vella L, Burton CZ, et al. Compensatory cognitive training for psychosis: effects in a randomized controlled trial. J Clin Psychiatry. 2012;73(9):1212–9.
190. Rispaud SG, Rose J, Kurtz MM. The relationship between change in cognition and change in functional ability in schizophrenia during cognitive and psychosocial rehabilitation. Psychiatry Res. 2016;244:145–50.
191. Kurtz MN, Moberg PJ, Gur RC, et al. Approaches to cognitive remediation of neuropsychological deficits in schizophrenia: a review and meta-analysis. Neuropsychol Rev. 2001;11(4):197–210.
192. Twamley EW, Jeste BV, Bellack AS. A review of cognitive training in schizophrenia. Schizophr Bull. 2003;29(2):359–82.
193. Pilling S, Bebbington P, Kuipers E, et al. Psychological treatments in schizophrenia: II. Meta-analyses of randomized controlled trials of social skills training and cognitive remediation. Psychol Med. 2002;32(5):783–91.
194. Grynszpan O, Perbal S, Pelissolo A, et al. Efficacy and specificity of computer-assisted cognitive remediation in schizophrenia: a meta-analytical study. Psychol Med. 2011;41(1):163–73.
195. Kurtz MM, Richardson CL. Social cognitive training for schizophrenia: a meta-analytic investigation of controlled research. Schizophr Bull. 2012;38(5):1092–104.
196. McGurk S, Twamley EW, Sitzer DI, et al. A meta-analysis of cognitive remediation in schizophrenia. Am J Psychiatry. 2007;164(12):1791–802.
197. Roder V, Mueller DR, Mueser KT, et al. Integrated psychological therapy (IPT) for schizophrenia: is it effective? Schizophr Bull. 2006;32(1):S81–93.
198. Roder V, Mueller DR, Schmidt SJ. Effectiveness of integrated psychological therapy (IPT) for schizophrenia patients: a research update. Schizophr Bull. 2011;37(2):S71–9.
199. Van Duin D, de Winter L, et al. The effect of rehabilitation combined with cognitive remediation on functioning in persons with severe mental illness: systematic review and meta-analysis. Psychol Med. 2019;49:1414–25.
200. Deste G, Barlati S, Cacciani P, et al. Persistence of effectiveness of cognitive remediation interventions in schizophrenia: a 1-year follow-up study. Schizophr Res. 2015;161(2–3):403–6.

201. Buonocore M, Spangaro M, Bechi M, et al. Integrated cognitive remediation and standard rehabilitation therapy in patients of schizophrenia: persistence after 5 years. Schizophr Res. 2018;192:335–9.
202. Cella M, Price T, Corboy H, et al. Cognitive remediation for inpatients with psychosis: a systematic review and meta-analysis. Psychol Med. 2020;50(7):1062–76.
203. Vita A, Barlati S, Ceraso A, et al. Effectiveness, Core Elements, and Moderators of Response of Cognitive Remediation for Schizophrenia: A Systematic Review and Meta-analysis of Randomized Clinical Trials. JAMA Psychiatry. 2021;78(8):848–58.
204. Prikken M, Konings MJ, et al. The efficacy of computerized cognitive drill and practice training for patients with a schizophrenia-spectrum disorder: a meta-analysis. Schizophr Res. 2019;204:368–74.
205. Kambeitz-Ilankovic L, Betz LT, Dominke C, et al. Multi-outcome meta-analysis (MOMA) of cognitive remediation in schizophrenia: revisiting the relevance of human coaching and elucidating interplay between multiple outcomes. Neurosci Biobehav Rev. 2019;107:828–45.
206. Yeh PY, Yu L, Guo NW, et al. Observation and imitation of social emotions are essential for improving cognitive and affective theory of mind in schizophrenia: a meta-analysis. J Nerv Ment Dis. 2019;207(6):474–81.
207. Lindenmayer JP, Khan A, McGurk SR, et al. Does social cognition training augment response to computer-assisted cognitive remediation for schizophrenia? Schizophr Res. 2018;201:180–6.
208. Abu-Akel A, Abushua'leh K. 'Theory of mind' in violent and nonviolent patients with paranoid schizophrenia. Schizophr Res. 2004;69:45–53.
209. Drury VM, Robinson EJ, Birchwood M. "Theory of mind" skills during an acute episode of psychosis and following recovery. Psychol Med. 1998;28:1101–12.
210. Greig TC, Bryson GJ, Bell MD. Theory of mind performance in schizophrenia: diagnostic, symptom, and neuropsychological correlates. J Nerv Ment Dis. 2004;192:12–8.
211. Pickup GJ, Frith CD. Theory of mind impairments in schizophrenia: symptomatology, severity and specificity. Psychol Med. 2001;31:207–20.
212. Grant N, Lawrence M, Preti A, et al. Social cognition interventions for people with schizophrenia: a systematic review focussing on methodological quality and intervention modality. Clin Psychol Rev. 2017;56:55–64.
213. Tan BL, Lee SA, Lee J. Social cognitive interventions for people with schizophrenia: a systematic review. Asian J Psychiatry. 2018;35:115–31.
214. Hong YY, Benet-Martinez V, Chiu CY, et al. Boundaries of cultural influence: construct activation as a mechanism for cultural differences in social perception. J Cross Cult Psychol. 2003;34:453–64.
215. Paquin K, Wilson AL, Cellard C, et al. A systematic review on improving cognition in schizophrenia: which is the more commonly used type of training, practice or strategy learning? BMC Psychiatry. 2014;14:139.
216. Roberts DL, Velligan DI. Can social functioning in schizophrenia be improved through targeted social cognitive intervention? Rehabil Res Pract. 2012;2012:742106.
217. Nijman SA, Veling W, et al. Social cognition training for people with a psychotic disorder: a network meta-analysis. Schizophr Bull. 2020;46(5):1086–103.
218. Farreny A, Aguado J, Corbera S, et al. Baseline predictors for success following strategy-based cognitive remediation group training in schizophrenia. J Nerv Ment Dis. 2016;204:585–9.
219. Barlati S, Deste G, Galluzzo A, et al. Factors associated with response and resistance to cognitive remediation in schizophrenia: a critical review. Front Pharmacol. 2019;9:1542.
220. Seccomandi B, Tsapekos D, Newbery K, et al. A systematic review of moderators of cognitive remediation response for people with schizophrenia. Schizophr Res Cogn. 2019;19:100160.
221. Barlati S, De Peri L, Deste G, et al. Cognitive remediation in the early course of schizophrenia: a critical review. Curr Pharm Des. 2012;18(4):534–41.
222. Edwards J, McGorry PD. Implementing early intervention in psychosis: a guide to establishing early psychosis services. London: Dunitz; 2002.
223. Keshavan MS, Hogarty GE. Brain maturational processes and delayed onset in schizophrenia. Dev Psychopathol. 1999;11(3):525–43.

224. McGorry PD, Edwards J, Mihalopoulos C, et al. EPPIC—an evolving system of early detection and optimal management. Schizophr Bull. 1996;22:305–26.
225. Killackey E. Psychosocial and psychological interventions in early psychosis: essential elements for recovery. Early Interv Psychiatry. 2009;3(1):S17–21.
226. Revell E, Neill JC, Harte M. A systematic review and meta-analysis of cognitive remediation in early schizophrenia. Schizophr Res. 2015;168:213–22.
227. Lewandowski KE. Cognitive remediation for the treatment of cognitive dysfunctions in the early course of psychosis. Harv Rev Psychiatry. 2016;24(2):164–72.
228. Devoe DJ, Farris MS, Townes P, et al. Interventions and social functioning in youth at risk of psychosis: a systematic review and meta-analysis. Early Interv Psychiatry. 2019;13(2):169–80.
229. Bellani M, Ricciardi C, Rossetti MG, et al. Cognitive remediation in schizophrenia: the earlier the better? Epidemiol Psychiatr Sci. 2019;29:e57.
230. Burns T. Evolution of outcome measures in schizophrenia. Br J Psychiatry Suppl. 2007;50:s1–6.
231. Juckel G, Morosini PL. The new approach: psychosocial functioning as a necessary outcome criterion for therapeutic success in schizophrenia. Curr Opin Psychiatry. 2008;21:630–9.
232. Priebe S. Social outcomes in schizophrenia. Br J Psychiatry. 2007;191:s15–20.
233. Karow A, Naber D. Subjective well-being and quality of life under atypical antipsychotic treatment. Psychopharmacology. 2002;162:3–10.
234. McGurk SR, Mueser KT. Cognitive functioning, symptoms, and work in supported employment: a review and heuristic model. Schizophr Res. 2004;70:147–74.
235. Mueser KT, Bellack AS, et al. Prediction of social skill acquisition in schizophrenic and major affective disorder patients from memory and symptomatology. Psychiatry Res. 1991;37:281–96.
236. Wykes T, Sturt E, Katz R. The prediction of rehabilitative success after three years—the use of social, symptom and cognitive variables. Br J Psychiatry. 1990;157:865–70.
237. Chan JYC, Hirai HW, Tsoi KKF. Can computer-assisted cognitive remediation improve employment and productivity outcomes of patients with severe mental illness? A meta-analysis of prospective controlled trials. J Psychiatr Res. 2015;68:293–300.
238. Pollice R, Roncone R, Falloon IRH, et al. Is theory of mind in schizophrenia more strongly associated with clinical and social functioning than with neurocognitive deficits? Psychopathology. 2002;35:280–8.
239. Brune M, Brune-Cohrs U. Theory of mind—evolution, ontogeny, brain mechanisms and psychopathology. Neurosci Biobehav Rev. 2006;30:437–55.
240. Robinson DG, Woerner MG, McMeniman M, et al. Symptomatic and functional recovery from a first episode of schizophrenia or schizoaffective disorder. Am J Psychiatry. 2004;161(3):473–9.
241. Butzlaff RL, Hooley JM. Expressed emotion and psychiatric relapse. Arch Gen Psychiatry. 1998;55:547–52.
242. Cella M, Preti A, Edwards C, et al. Cognitive remediation for negative symptoms of schizophrenia: a network meta-analysis. Clin Psychol Rev. 2017;52:43–51.
243. Cella M, Stahl D, Morris S, et al. Effects of cognitive remediation on negative symptoms dimensions exploring the role of working memory. Psychol Med. 2017;47:2593–601.
244. Fusar-Poli P, Papanastasiou E, Stahl D, et al. Treatments of negative symptoms in schizophrenia: meta-analysis of 168 randomized placebo-controlled trials. Schizophr Bull. 2015;41(4):892–9.
245. Bowie CR, Bell MD, Fiszdon JM, et al. Cognitive remediation for schizophrenia: an expert working group white paper on core techniques. Schizophr Res. 2020;215:49–53.
246. Penadés R, Franck N, González-Vallespí L, Dekerle M. Neuroimaging studies of cognitive function in schizophrenia. Adv Exp Med Biol. 2019;1118:117–34.

Psychotic Disorders and Substance Abuse Comorbidity: Characteristics and Treatment

3

Kirsten Catthoor and Geert Dom

3.1 Introduction

Recently, there is a tendency to use a more dimensionally based conceptualization of psychopathology to describe psychosis instead of the traditional medical model of categorical diagnosis. Psychosis is described as a stage of heightened awareness and emotionality combined with a sense of anxiety and impasse, in an overstimulated brain that is not able to filter incoming stimuli properly [1]. The main reason for this paradigm shift is that schizophrenia represents only the 30% poor outcome of a much broader spectrum of psychotic disorders [2]. Clinicians, researchers, and advocacy groups plead to implement a psychosis spectrum disorder because much remains to be clarified in terms of etiology, diagnosis, and treatment [2]. From a classical psychiatric perspective, psychosis is a continuum-based syndrome with positive, negative, cognitive, mood, and motor symptoms. Patients with psychosis have a unique pattern of symptoms that can change over time. In acute illness, positive symptoms are predominantly present, while negative, affective, and cognitive symptoms are responsible for difficulties in daily life during periods of recovery.

Positive symptoms are called "positive" because they add a surplus of mental experiences that were not present before. They include hallucinations and delusions. Hallucinations are sensory experiences without a neurological pathway from the senses to the brain. Hearing voices is the most common and well-known

K. Catthoor
Collaborative Antwerp Psychiatric Research Institute (CAPRI), Antwerp University (UA), Antwerp, Belgium

ZNA Stuivenberg, Antwerp, Belgium
e-mail: kirsten.catthoor@zna.be

G. Dom (✉)
Collaborative Antwerp Psychiatric Research Institute (CAPRI), Antwerp University (UA), Antwerp, Belgium
e-mail: geert.dom@uantwerpen.be

P. Rocca, S. Bellino (eds.), *Psychosis and Personality Disorders*,
https://doi.org/10.1007/978-3-031-09058-5_3

example. However, all our five senses can be implicated, e.g., smelling fire, seeing threatening monsters, and feeling bugs under the skin are among other possible hallucinatory perceptions. Delusions are inadequate thoughts and persuasions for which there are no firm arguments in reality. Paranoia, the conviction of being in great danger and nowhere to be safe, being followed or persecuted affects the majority of patients. Besides, delusional convictions can include content of grandiosity, religiosity, and hypochondria. Positive symptoms are hypothetically linked to malfunctions in the mesolimbic brain circuit [3].

The negative symptom domain contains anhedonia, asociality, avolition, blunted affect, and alogia. Negative symptoms are called "negative" because they express a lack of features or a withdrawal of behavior, compared with the premorbid condition. Anhedonia is experiencing difficulties in feeling pleasure during social, recreational, or physical activities. Asociality can be understood as a clearly reduced social activity, together with a decreased interest in forming close relationships with other people. Avolition means the reduction in initiating activities or persisting in doing them. Patients with blunted affect show a marked decrease in facial and vocational expression of emotions. Alogia contains aspects of reduced quantity of speech, and spontaneous elaboration during a conversation. Some research emphasized disturbances in dopaminergic and noradrenergic circuitry, related to the ventral striatum reward system as neural substrates for the negative symptoms of psychosis. Other studies endorse alterations in both dorsal and ventral corticostriatal systems, and alterations in normal connectivity among brain regions [4].

Working memory problems, attention and concentration deficits, and limitations in learning new information and in executive functioning are among the most prominent neurocognitive impairments in psychosis. They are linked to dysfunctional dopamine and N-methyl-D-aspartate interactions in the prefrontal cortex and altered glutamatergic neurotransmitter pathways in the hippocampus. Cognitive performance is a firm predictor of global functioning in daily life for patients with psychosis [5].

Affective and depressive symptoms are highly prevalent in middle-aged and older persons with psychosis [6]. Persons with psychosis report significantly higher real-time depressed mood than the healthy controls and also indicate significantly higher retrospective depressive feelings [7].

In line with affective problems, suicidal ideation, suicide attempts, and completion are frequently associated with a diagnosis of psychotic disorder. The lifetime suicide rate in individuals with schizophrenia is approximately 10% [8]. Of importance, the rate of suicide seems to decrease (OR 0.52) in periods of antipsychotic medication use versus periods of medication noncompliance [9]. In contrast to the relative beneficial effect of pharmacotherapy, a co-occurring substance use disorder significantly increases the risk on suicidality within individuals with psychosis. The risk of suicide attempts and completed suicide in patients with schizophrenia with a SUD versus without a SUD is, respectively, OR 3.41 and OR 2.6 [10].

Recently, psychomotor slowing has been added to the core symptoms of psychosis. It is characterized by the slowing of planning, initiation, and execution of movements. Psychomotor slowing can be differentiated from negative symptoms because of the absence of an association between planning and execution and negative symptoms [11].

The recent World Mental Health Surveys of the World Health Organization [12] endorses the importance of co-occurring substance use and psychosis. It showed frequent bidirectional associations between psychotic experiences and substance use and substance use disorders. Although not all types of substances are associated with psychotic experiences, it is important to keep the possibility in mind, when confronted with patients in clinical mental health practice. In this study, lifetime tobacco use, extra-medical prescription drug use, alcohol use, and alcohol use disorders were associated with a higher risk of developing psychotic experiences even after controlling for potential confounding factors. Similarly, preceding psychotic experiences were associated with subsequent onset of tobacco, alcohol, and cannabis use, and all substance use disorders. To predict substance use disorders among substance users, only the associations between psychotic experiences and alcohol disorders remained significant after adjusting for antecedent mental disorders.

3.2 Epidemiology

An updated systematic review on the prevalence of psychosis by Moreno-Küstner and Martín [13], revealed a 12-month prevalence for people with psychosis of 4.03 per 1000 and a median lifetime prevalence of 7.49 per 1000. Not remarkably, psychosis in the general population showed higher prevalence rates than in mental health care and/or social services. The CAMFEPS study describes a total yearly incidence of first episode psychosis of 34.1 per 10.0000 per annum in a naturalistic mental health care network [14]. In any DSM-IV diagnostic criterium of psychotic disease, men were 1.30 times more affected than women. In this study, substance-induced psychotic disorder was primarily a disorder of younger males in association with a wide range of substances.

The use of substances is highly prevalent within many societies. In many (Western) countries, up to 80% of the adult population uses or has used alcohol. Next to alcohol, the use of cannabis is high in many countries. The European Monitoring Centre for Drugs and Drug Addiction estimates the use of cannabis in 2019 as much of 7.4% of the total population. The lifetime use comes close to 27.4%. For young adults (aged between 15 and 34 years) the percentage of users approaches 14.4%.

Substance use disorders (SUDs) are among the most common psychiatric disorders and are responsible for a major proportion of morbidity, sickness absenteeism, and mortality in the population. In Europe and the United States alcohol use disorders (with a lifetime and annual prevalence in the population of 13% and 4%, respectively), for instance, occupy fifth place as regards the number of years of life lost (adjusted for quality of life), with only ischemic heart disease, cerebrovascular disorders, depressive disorder, and dementia coming higher in Europe. Smoking (lifetime prevalence in the population 22%) is at the same time the main cause of premature death, being responsible for approximately 14% of all deaths in 2001. The number of people addicted to illegal substances (drugs)—lifetime prevalence in the population of 6%—is much smaller than the number of alcohol and tobacco addicts, and the effects on people's state of health are much less.

3.3 Psychosis and (Ab)use of Substances

A Norwegian population study [15] showed an incidence of 6.5 persons per 100.000 for a first episode substance-induced psychosis, and 9.7 per 100.00 for psychotic patients misusing substances. The incidence for persons with psychosis, but not misusing substances, was 24.1 per 100.000. Patient characteristics for first episode substance-induced psychosis were short duration of untreated psychosis, male preponderance, more positive symptoms at baseline, and poorer premorbid academic achievements in early adolescence. In Denmark [16], the incidence of cannabis-induced psychosis more than doubled from 2.8 per 100.000 person years in 2006, to 6.1 in 2016. Dual diagnosis of schizophrenia and cannabis use disorder increased in a corresponding way. The same study showed a corresponding decrease in alcohol-induced psychosis, from 5 per 100.000 to less than 2.

A systematic review and meta-analysis on comorbid substance use in patients with schizophrenia spectrum disorders in community and clinical settings revealed that substance use is highly prevalent in this population [17]. Large surveys show that the prevalence of SUD in individuals with schizophrenia is between 47% and 44%. The most frequently used substances are alcohol and cannabis. In addition, between 60 and 90% of individuals with schizophrenia or psychosis are tobacco dependent [18]. Rates did not change substantially over time and men were more affected than women. Patients with substance use showed earlier onset of the psychotic disorder, compared to nonusers.

3.3.1 Psychosis and Cannabis

There is not a single doubt that patients with psychosis use cannabis more often, compared to the general population. It has been scientifically proven, and published in many papers, in different countries around the globe. On the other hand, psychosis has been connected to many other risk factors and cannabis is just one of them. In a critical review on the relationship between psychosis and cannabis, Ksir and Hart [19] suggest three models of causality. The diathesis-stress model emphasizes a variety of genetic, gestational, infectious, nutritional, and toxic factors like substances to increase the vulnerability to psychosis. In the causal model, cannabis plays an essential role as an environmental stressor which leads directly to the appearance of psychotic behavior. Besides, the shared vulnerability hypothesis enhances the chances of both cannabis use and psychosis. Early and heavy cannabis use may be considered as one of several prodromal signs predicting an increasing risk for developing psychosis. A meta-analysis by Murrie [20] on the transition from substance-induced psychosis to schizophrenia, revealed cannabis as the most predictive factor. Thirty-four percent of people with cannabis-induced psychosis developed schizophrenia later in life, based on a cohort of 3400 patients in six studies.

In the largest genome wide association study on lifetime cannabis use [21] a range of correlations suggests that genetic liability to lifetime cannabis use should be considered within a broader context of personality and mental health traits. The substantial genetic correlations with risk-taking behavior and craving for experience may indicate that the tendency to experiment with cannabis is a trait of one's personality. The authors indicate that there is weak evidence that cannabis use leads to the development of schizophrenia, but there are many more scientific arguments that people susceptible to developing schizophrenia will seek out the use of cannabis. This suggests that individuals with a higher liability to schizophrenia have a higher risk to start using cannabis.

Another recent study on genetics [22] found a supplementary effect of molecular genetic risk state for schizophrenia with the presence of lifetime regular cannabis use and exposure to early-life adversities like sexual abuse, emotional abuse, emotional neglect, and bullying. The authors considered the combined influence of genetic liability and environmental exposure as larger than the sum of the individual risk components.

Cannabis use is responsible for a substantial amount of psychosis-related hospital admissions. Trends are even increasing [23]. Data from the USA, France, and Portugal warrant policy makers for legalizing cannabis for recreational use [16, 23]. In Portugal, where the possession of cannabis for personal use was decriminalized in 2001, hospital admissions for psychotic episodes linked to cannabis use, multiplied by a factor 29.4 from 2000 to 2015. The increasing numbers of hospitalizations, despite deinstitutionalization in mental health care, could be explained by higher consumer patterns, higher potency of the cannabis, and patients of average younger age.

Taken together, as reviewed by a recent "review of reviews" the scientific literature indicates that psychotic illness arises more frequently in cannabis users compared to nonusers, cannabis use is associated with a dose-dependent risk of developing psychotic illness, and cannabis users have an earlier onset of psychotic illness compared to nonusers. Cannabis use was also associated with increased relapse rates, more hospitalizations, and pronounced positive symptoms in psychotic patients [24].

3.3.2 Psychosis and (Met)Amphetamines

According to a review from the Lancet [25] on global stimulant use, amphetamine dependence was associated with 1–23% of suicide deaths, 0–59% of accidental injury deaths, 0–48% of cardiovascular deaths, and 1–23% of homicide deaths in 2017. The use of stimulants appears to be a major challenge for general and mental health care worldwide. Murrie [20] found a transition rate of 22% from amphetamine-induced psychosis to schizophrenia.

A recent, very well-executed review and meta-analysis revealed that any use of amphetamines was associated with a doubled risk of developing psychosis [26]. An amphetamine use disorder tripled the risk. Most evidence was derived from high-quality cross-sectional studies. Besides, there is evidence from longitudinal studies for a dose-related increase in psychotic symptoms during amphetamine using periods. More psychotic disorders are associated with amphetamine use disorders when compared to other substance use disorders except for cannabis use.

The same high prevalence of psychotic features was found in a population of methamphetamine use disorder patients. More severe drug use problems, emotional symptoms, and cognitive impairment were reported in a large sample of methamphetamine use disorder patients [27]. Earlier onset of drug use, higher quantity of drug use, higher craving, middle or severe drug use disorder, and a higher amount of anxiety symptoms were established as the main associated risk factors for developing methamphetamine use-induced psychotic disorder.

Special attention is needed for persons with ADHD who receive treatment for this with amphetamines or methylphenidate. Moran [28] found an incidence of a psychotic episode of 1.78 per 1000 patients taking methylphenidate and 2.83 per 1000 persons who were treated with amphetamines. The higher risk for psychosis with amphetamines compared to methylphenidate can be explained by the different biological interactions between both drugs and the neurotransmitter metabolism in the brain. Approximately 1 in 660 patients who received a prescription for stimulants for ADHD, will develop a first onset psychosis because of this.

3.3.3 Psychosis and Alcohol

Alcohol-induced psychotic disorder is a DSM-5 classified psychiatric disorder resulting from a chronic alcohol use disorder. The main symptoms of the syndrome include delusions, hallucinations, usually in the form of derogatory and threatening voices, affective problems, impaired cognitive processing, and inappropriate behavior [29]. An alcohol-induced psychotic disorder is clearly distinct from an alcohol withdrawal delirium: delusions are better organized versus incoherent; hallucinations are mostly verbal-auditory versus visual (small moving objects like insects), and a higher intensity of fearful affect [30]. The same paper mentioned a lower level of education in patients with alcohol-induced psychotic disorder, later origin of the psychotic symptoms, a higher level of anxiety and depressive symptoms, less negative symptoms, a better insight into the mental problems, and less functional decline.

From an epidemiologic point of view [30], a point prevalence of alcohol-induced psychotic disorder is estimated between 0.4% and 0.6% in patients hospitalized for alcohol use disorder, and a lifetime prevalence of 7.5% in the same population. Lifetime prevalence in the general population is 0.41% versus 0.18% for alcohol withdrawal delirium. The highest lifetime prevalence is found in males between 45 and 54 years old. A Swedish population study [31] showed the cumulative risk for progression to schizophrenia from any substance-induced psychotic disorder was 11.3%, but the lowest for alcohol-induced psychotic disorder.

Patients with alcohol-induced psychotic disorder had a higher healthcare utilization (50%-increase per annum) compared with age, sex, and general practice-matched control population before the diagnosis was officially set [29]. The excess can be explained by a higher prevalence of alcohol-related morbidities in patients, like alcohol-specific conditions (alcoholic liver damage, alcoholic cardiomyopathy, alcohol-induced chronic pancreatitis, alcoholic gastritis, alcoholic polyneuropathy, etc.) and alcohol-related conditions (oral cancers, esophageal cancer, ischemic heart disease, injuries, interpersonal violence, etc.). Seizures and injuries (both intentional and unintentional) were more strongly associated with later development of alcoholic psychosis. Assaults and self-harm were accountable for more than 80% of the injury burden among patients.

3.3.4 Psychosis and Tobacco

Tobacco smoking is known to be harmful to physical health in many different ways. It is the leading cause of preventable death. It increases the risk of cancer, chronic obstructive pulmonary disease, coronary heart disease, cerebrovascular disease, asthma, and diabetes. There is evidence that nicotine alters signaling in the dopaminergic, cholinergic, and glutamatergic neurotransmitter systems in the adolescent brain. Nicotine use in vulnerable periods during adolescence could disrupt brain maturation [32].

Smoking rates in individuals with mental illness are approximately double compared to adults without mental disorders [33]. More than half of the entire nicotine use worldwide is used by patients with psychiatric problems. Mental illness is associated with higher levels of nicotine dependence, intensity of smoking, and smoking severity. Besides, there is less success in attempts to stop smoking. The high prevalence of smoking in patients with psychiatric disorders was explained by the self-medication hypothesis for many years. This assumption postulates that patients with psychosis derive symptomatic relief of cognitive decline and side effects of antipsychotic medication and a higher quality of life. A study on cognition in patients with first episode psychosis and its association with tobacco smoking (2018) [34] could not support this. The results did not show any significant difference between smokers and non-smokers in verbal memory, visual memory, working memory, processing speed, executive function, motor dexterity and attention, independent of gender, age, education, or premorbid IQ. Vermeulen [35] also disputes the self-medication hypothesis in a large prospective, longitudinal cohort study. Smoking patients with psychotic disorder, as well as their siblings and healthy controls showed more symptoms than their nonsmoking counterparts. Patients who quit smoking did not develop a worsening symptom tableau compared to those who did not change their smoking behavior. Also, starting to smoke or increasing the number of cigarettes did not weaken symptoms; on the contrary, patients reported higher symptom frequency.

Two systematic reviews and meta-analyses have examined the association between tobacco smoking and psychotic disorders. Both report a twofold risk for psychotic disorders in heavy smoking people [36, 37]. Scott [38] found six out of eight studies on psychosis and tobacco to report a positive association between tobacco smoking and risk of developing a psychotic disorder, using causal criteria of the Bradford Hill Framework Hill. The authors of this study emphasize the association between tobacco smoking and psychotic disorders warrants further attention, especially with higher availability and use of e-cigarettes in adolescence. Mustonen [32] confirms heavy tobacco smoking as an independent risk factor for psychosis even after adjustment for a range of confounders in adolescents.

3.4 Mechanisms Underlying Comorbidity

Different mechanisms may contribute to the increased risk of psychosis—SUD Comorbidity. These different pathways, combined or single, may or may not play a role within an individual patient development.

3.4.1 Auto-Medication

Initially, the auto-medication hypothesis finds its origin in psychoanalytical theories, which postulated that drugs are used as a coping mechanism against psychotic aggressive tendencies. Other authors hypothesize that neuroleptic dysphoria is likely the missing link between schizophrenia and substance abuse. Medication-induced dysphoria could possibly play a significant role in the development of drug comorbidity in schizophrenia and related psychoses [39]. Recently, neurobiological support for the self-medication hypothesis was integrated in the existing theories [39]. Low striatal dopamine does not only inflict neuroleptic-induced dysphoria, but also provokes comorbid vulnerability to addictive states. It should be clear, however, that the abovementioned recent genetic research revealed evidence for the opposite direction of causality [21].

3.4.2 Early Childhood Adversity

Increasing evidence emphasizes the strong association between early child maltreatment and severe mental illness later in life, including psychosis. Epidemiological data also show high levels of comorbidity between psychosis and other mental health problems, like substance use. A narrative review and meta-analysis [40] revealed that childhood adversity and trauma substantially increase the risk of psychosis with an OR of 2.8. All types of adversity were related to an increased risk of psychosis, but there was no evidence that any specific type of trauma was a stronger predictor of psychosis. Noteworthy, the risk of developing psychosis following childhood trauma is most probably independent of that assigned by cannabis exposure.

A large Australian epidemiological study [41] investigated the association between childhood adversity experiences in psychotic patients and clinical mental health features and psychosocial outcomes. Patients reporting any form of childhood adversity showed higher social dysfunction. More victimization and offending were found, but the strongest association was for homelessness. From a clinical point of view, associations with depression, self-harm, and suicidal thoughts were commonly present. Associations between any childhood adversity and hallucinations and subjective thought disorder were found, but not delusions. Hallucinations were strongly associated with childhood sexual abuse. In line with other studies, an association between any form of childhood adversity and alcohol and other substance dependence was distinct.

3.4.3 Common Underlying Neurobiological Factors

Although the neurobiological aspects relevant to the pathogenesis of both SUD and psychosis are still far from revealed, similar dysfunctions in neurobiological systems, circuitries, and their associated functional effects, might make individuals vulnerable to both psychosis and SUD development. Khokhar et al. [42] propose a unifying hypothesis based upon recent evidence from epidemiological and genetic association studies with brain imaging and preclinical studies. They suggest that the genetic determinants of risk for schizophrenia (especially within neural systems that contribute to the risk for both psychosis and addiction) make patients vulnerable to substance use. Since this vulnerability may arise prior to the appearance of psychotic symptoms, an increased use of substances in adolescence may both enhance the risk for developing a later substance use disorder, and also serve as an additional risk factor for the appearance of psychotic symptoms[42, 43].

3.5 Screening and Diagnosis on SUD

Given the high prevalence of substance use and misuse within individuals with psychosis, standard screening, and if positive assessment, on SUD should be mandatory in every treatment context. Different screening instruments are available, although it needs to be noted that none of these instruments have been validated within individuals with psychosis. However, it can be estimated that, outside of the acute psychotic episode, these instruments can be used with a validity (specificity, sensitivity) that is comparable with other populations.

Various screening tools are available to identify use disorders, namely brief questionnaires for general practice that can be completed quickly. The best-known are:

- The Cut down, Annoyed, Guilty, Eye-opener (CAGE)
- Substance Abuse Screening Tool
- The Alcohol Use Disorders Identification Test (AUDIT)
- The Derived Alcohol Use Disorders Identification Test (AUDIT-C)
- The Drug Abuse Screening Test (DAST) for drug problems
- The Fagerström Test for Nicotine Dependence (FTND) for tobacco addiction

(http://ndri.curtin.edu.au/btitp/documents/Fagerstrom_test.pdf).

Physical examination and laboratory tests can sometimes provide clues when trying to identify current drug use and the physical effects of prolonged excessive use. The products themselves (and their metabolites) can be detected using various laboratory techniques on various samples (urine, hair, blood), and certain abnormal blood values can be measured that are somewhat specific (but by no means entirely) to the effects of alcohol.

Both screeners, physical examination and laboratory tests can provide clues that can assist in diagnosis, but ultimately a diagnosis of "substance use disorder" can only be made based on interviewing the patient, and information from those around the patient (history through an informant) is often essential.

3.6 Treatment

3.6.1 General Aspects

Comorbidity of SUD within individuals with psychosis has an overall negative impact on prognosis, in part driven by a serious negative impact on treatment compliance.

3.6.2 Psychosocial Interventions

A recent Cochrane review (Dec 2019) consisting of 41 trials with a total of 4024 participants, revealed no constraining evidence for psychosocial treatments to reduce either substance abuse or diminish mental health symptoms in patients with dual diagnosis (https://www.cochrane.org/CD001088/SCHIZ_psychosocial-interventions-people-both-severe-mental-illness-and-substance-misuse). The methodological quality of most of the studies was rather limited. Motivational interviewing provided modest positive effects on patients restraining from alcohol and attending the first aftercare appointment. In combination with cognitive behavioral therapy, it can also improve mental health state, life satisfaction, and social functioning. The authors suggest mental health professionals to keep up with recent scientific findings that could rapidly provide evidence for particular forms of treatment.

In November 2016, the National Institute for Health and Care Excellence (NICE) published guidelines on community health and social care services for coexisting severe mental illness and substance misuse in general (https://www.nice.org.uk/guidance/ng58/chapter/Recommendations). For psychosis and substance use, in particular, NICE guidelines were developed in 2011 (https://www.nice.org.uk/guidance/cg120/chapter/Introduction). General recommendations are attention to the multiple needs of this vulnerable patient group, like physical health problems, homelessness, unstable housing, and stigma. Meeting the safeguarding needs of all people with coexisting severe mental illness and substance misuse, and their carers and wider family are emphasized. Deontological considerations on referral to secondary mental health care services are mentioned: not to exclude patients with serious mental illness because of their substance misuse, and not restrain them from care. A person-centered approach is to be adopted. In secondary mental health care, a personal care plan is developed in collaboration with the patient and his relatives, based on his strengths and possibilities, and taking into account his vulnerabilities. The care plan should be a multiagency approach to address physical health, social care, housing, and other support needs. For the organization of care, partnership between specialist services, health, social care, and other support services and commissioners is needed.

NICE guidelines for persons with psychosis and concomitant substance misuse enhance the importance of offering evidence-based treatments for both conditions. Ineffective treatments should be discontinued, effective treatments must be acceptable for the person involved. Complex and individual relationships between substance misuse, psychotic symptoms, emotional state, behavior, and the person's social context have to be taken into account. A treatment plan for a person with psychosis and coexisting substance misuse and the sequencing of treatments should be tailored to the relative severity of both the psychosis and the substance misuse at different times, the person's social and treatment context, and the person's readiness for change. Inpatient mental health facilities should ensure that they have policies and procedures for promoting a therapeutic environment free from drugs and alcohol and provide them soon after the admission. These should include search procedures, visiting arrangements, planning and reviewing leave, drug and alcohol testing, disposal of legal and illicit substances, and other security measures.

Psychosocial treatment approaches to psychosis, which also address the destructive consequences of adverse childhood events, are likely to be effective for many patients. It is very important to make them available and accessible [44].

3.6.3 Pharmacological Aspects

3.6.3.1 Antipsychotic Medications

NICE guidelines (https://www.nice.org.uk/guidance/cg120/chapter/Introduction) state there is no evidence for any differential benefit for one antipsychotic over another for people with psychosis and coexisting substance misuse. A random effects meta-analysis on efficacy, acceptability, and tolerability of antipsychotics in patients with schizophrenia and comorbid substance use [45] showed clozapine to be superior to other antipsychotics for reduction of substance use. Risperidone reduced craving more than olanzapine. Olanzapine, clozapine, and risperidone showed superiority for symptom reduction compared to other drugs. Results of side effects followed known patterns but were not always reported.

Psychotic patients with co-occurrent drug abuse may be more sensitive to the extrapyramidal, cardiovascular, and metabolic side effects of antipsychotics [46]. Choosing antipsychotic agents proven based on their side effect profile is warranted for this population of patients.

A survey of Italian psychiatrists and other clinicians on clinical management of psychotic patients with substance use [47] revealed they consider substance use to be a serious complicating factor in mental health care treatment. In the acute setting, haloperidol was used as the first-line agent of choice followed by aripiprazole and olanzapine. In the maintenance phase, aripiprazole was the dominantly used first-line agent, followed by olanzapine. Half of the responding clinicians used long-acting agents.

3.6.3.2 Medications Used for Substance Abuse Treatment

Pharmacological treatments are available for the treatment of alcohol, heroin, and nicotine addiction. Studies show a moderate (alcohol, heroin) to weak (nicotine) effectivity in comparison with placebo. Although most of these studies have been done within individuals without major psychiatric comorbidity, the limited number of studies within patients with psychosis or schizophrenia suggest that these medications can be used safely and effectively within these comorbid patient groups.

Treatment of Alcohol Use Disorders

Several studies have examined the safety and efficacy of medications (i.e., naltrexone, disulfiram, and acamprosate) used to treat AUD in individuals with co-occurring schizophrenia and AUD [48, 49]. Different (albeit mostly small studies) show a reduction of fewer drinking days, less heavy drinking days, and less craving in patients with schizophrenia.

Theoretically, disulfiram has a risk of worsening psychosis in predisposed individuals because of its action of inhibiting dopamine beta-hydroxylase, but this phenomenon appears to be rare in clinical practice [50]. In a small study, disulfiram was well tolerated and found beneficial in patients with schizophrenia [51]. Supervision (by staff or family) over disulfiram intake is mandatory in view of effectivity. In addition, the use of disulfiram is contraindicated for patients with cardiovascular or hepatic problems.

Taken together, although few studies have been done within patients with schizophrenia, naltrexone, and acamprosate can be safely used to treat co-morbid AUD in patients with schizophrenia.

Smoking

In a very comprehensive guidance document, smoking and mental health, the Royal College of Physicians stress the evidence and need [52] for smoking cessation programs in patients with serious mental illness, including psychosis. Different studies show that varenicline, bupropion, and nicotine substitution (patches) can be used safely and effectively by individuals with schizophrenia, as a treatment for nicotine dependence [53, 54] Peckham [54]. Remarkably, people with psychosis can counter smoking habits with the same interventions that work for people in the general population. Recently there is some evidence that E(electronic) cigarettes have a similar effect on the quit rate as NRT, but this topic deserves further research. First studies show that also within individuals with a psychiatric comorbidity E-cigarettes might be a valuable option in view of smoking reduction and cessation [55].

Opiate Use Disorders

Interestingly heroin and by extension all opioid substances have a (weak) antipsychotic effect. However, severe heroin addiction seems to be rare in patients with schizophrenia. Opioid maintenance therapy is among the most effective treatments within the addiction field, specifically aiming at improving treatment adherence and reducing risks associated with heroin use; i.e., medical (hepatitis, AIDS), legal (criminal acts), and social (re-enabling work). The most frequently used pharmacological treatments in MT are all opioid agonists; methadone and buprenorphine. Different, small-scaled, studies indicate that both can be used within patients with schizophrenia [56]. However, the prescription and follow-up of opioid (agonist) maintenance therapy need to be in the hands of a trained (addiction) doctor, given the specificities of these treatments. Among others, caution needs to be taken, since both methadone (and heroin) can cause QT-prolongation, risks that should be evaluated specifically in view of concomitant use of antipsychotic medication.

Taken together, although more studies are needed, the current research evidence and clinical experience suggest that when treating co-morbid substance abuse within patients with schizophrenia, the same pharmacological strategies can be used that are included in the guidelines for treatment of "addiction only" patients.

3.6.4 Organizational Aspects

Crockford and Addington [18] published Canadian guidelines on schizophrenia and other psychotic disorders with coexisting substance use disorders by integrating different guidelines that were assembled after 2010. Recommendations of the National Institute for Health and Care Excellence (NICE), the Scottish Intercollegiate Guidelines Network (SIGN), the American Psychiatric Association, the American Academy of Child and Adolescent Psychiatry, and the European Psychiatric Association were integrated in their text. In the organization of care, the management of all persons with psychosis and coexisting substance use disorders should be based on a comprehensive, multidisciplinary assessment. Integrated substance use and psychosis treatment provided in the same mental health care setting is considered to offer the best treatment outcomes compared with care provided in a parallel or sequential fashion. Unfortunately, integrated care is limited availability.

3.7 Conclusions

The frequent comorbidity of schizophrenia and SUD is associated with negative long-term outcomes. The integrated treatment approach should focus on long-term, motivation based, both psychosis and substance-use specialized mental health care treatment programs because they have some proven advantages over standard care. Unfortunately, integrated treatment programs are expensive and in many countries not sufficiently available. Careful development of inpatient, outpatient, and outreach treatment modalities and guidelines for different subgroups of patients is an urgent matter in modern mental health care.

References

1. Kapur S. Psychosis as a state of aberrant salience: a framework linking biology, phenomenology, and pharmacology in schizophrenia. Am J Psychiatry. 2003;160(1):13–23.
2. Guloksuz S, van Os J. The slow death of the concept of schizophrenia and the painful birth of the psychosis spectrum. Psychol Med. 2018;48(2):229–44.
3. Keshavan M, Collin G, Guimond S, Kelly S, Prasad K, Lizano P. Neuroimaging in Schizophrenia. Neuroimaging Clin N Am. 2020;30(1):73–83.
4. Stepien M, Manoliu A, Kubli R, Schneider K, Tobler P, Seifritz E, Herdener M, Kaiser S, Kirschner M. Investigating the association of ventral and dorsal striatal dysfunction during reward anticipation with negative symptoms in patients with schizophrenia and healthy individuals. PLoS One. 2018;13(6):e0198215.
5. McCleerey A, Nuechterlein K. Cognitive impairment in psychotic illness: prevalence, profile of impairment, developmental course, and treatment considerations. Dialogues Clin Neurosci. 2019;21(3):239–48.
6. Zisook S, Nyer M, Kasckow J, Golshan S, Lehman D, Montross L. Depressive symptom patterns in patients with chronic schizophrenia and subsyndromal depression. Schizophr Res. 2006;86(1–3):226–33.
7. Blum L, Vakhrusheva J, Saperstein A, Khan S, Chang R, Hansen M, Zemon V, Kimhyb D. Depressed mood in individuals with schizophrenia: A comparison of retrospective and real-time measures. Psychiatry Res. 2015;227(0):318–23.
8. Sher L, Kahn R. Suicide in schizophrenia: an educational overview. Medicina (Kaunas). 2019;55(7) https://doi.org/10.3390/medicina55070361.
9. Taipale H, Tanskanen A, Mehtala J, Vattulainen P, Correll C, Tiihonen J. 20-year follow-up study of physical morbidity and mortality in relationship to antipsychotic treatment in a nationwide cohort of 62,250 patients with schizophrenia (FIN20). World Psychiatry. 2020;19(1):61–8. https://doi.org/10.1002/wps.20699.
10. Ostergaard M, Nordentoft M, Hjorthoj C. Associations between substance use disorders and suicide or suicide attempts in people with mental illness: a Danish nation-wide, prospective, register-based study of patients diagnosed with schizophrenia, bipolar disorder, unipolar depression or personality disorder. Addiction. 2017;112(7):1250–9. https://doi.org/10.1111/add.13788.
11. Bervoets C, Docx L, Sabbe B, Vermeulen S, Van Den Bossche M, Morsel A, Morrens M. The nature of the relationship of psychomotor slowing with negative symptomatology in schizophrenia. Cogn Neuropsychiatry. 2014;19(1):36–46. https://doi.org/10.1080/13546805.2013.779578.
12. Degenhardt L, Saha S, Lim C, Aguilar-Gaxiola S, Al-Hamzawi A, Alonso J, Andrade L, Bromet E, Bruffaerts R, et al. The associations between psychotic experiences and substance use and substance use disorders: findings from the World Health Organization world mental health surveys. Addiction. 2018;113(5):924–34.
13. Moreno-Küstner B, Martín C, Pastor L. Prevalence of psychotic disorders and its association with methodological issues. A systematic review and meta-analyses. PLoS One. 2018;13(4):e0195687.
14. Nkire N, Scully P, Browne D, Baldwin P, Kingston T, Owoeye O, Kinsella A, O'Callaghan E, Russell V, Waddington L. Systematic epidemiological and clinical comparisons across all 12 DSM-IV psychotic diagnoses in the Cavan-Monaghan first episode psychosis study (CAMFEPS). Psychol Med. 2019;20:1–10.

15. Weibell M, Jørgen Bramness I, Johannessen J, McGorry P, ten Velden Hegelstad W, Ketil Larsen T. Treated incidence and baseline characteristics of substance induced psychosis in a Norwegian catchment area. BMC Psychiatry. 2013;27(13):319.
16. Hjorthøj C, Larsen M, Starzer M, Nordentoft M. Annual incidence of cannabis-induced psychosis, other substance-induced psychoses and dually diagnosed schizophrenia and cannabis use disorder in Denmark from 1994 to 2016. Psychol Med. 2019 Dec;16:1–6.
17. Hunt G, Large M, Cleary M, Lai H, Saunders J. Prevalence of comorbid substance use in schizophrenia spectrum disorders in community and clinical settings, 1990-2017: systematic review and meta-analysis. Drug Alcohol Depend. 2018;1(191):234–58.
18. Crockford D, Addington D. Canadian schizophrenia guidelines: schizophrenia and other psychotic disorders with coexisting substance use disorders. Can J Psychiatr. 2017;62(9):624–34. https://doi.org/10.1177/0706743717720196.
19. Ksir C, Hart C. Cannabis and psychosis: a critical overview of the relationship. Curr Psychiatry Rep. 2016;18(2):12.
20. Murrie B, Lappin J, Large M, Sara G. Transition of substance-induced, brief, and atypical psychoses to schizophrenia: a systematic review and meta-analysis. Schizophr Bull. 2019;46(3):505–16.
21. Pasman J, Verweij K, Gerring Z, Stringer S, Sanchez-Roige S, Treur J, Abdellaoui A, Nivard M, et al. GWAS of lifetime cannabis use reveals new risk loci, genetic overlap with psychiatric traits, and a causal effect of schizophrenia liability. Nat Neurosci. 2018;21:1161–70.
22. Guloksuz S, Pries L-K, Delespaul P, Kenis G, Luykx J, Lin B, Richards A, Akdede B. … Van Os, J. examining the independent and joint effects of molecular genetic liability and environmental exposures in schizophrenia: results from the EUGEI study. World Psychiatry. 2019;18:173–82.
23. Gonçalves-Pinho M, Bragança M, Freitas A. Psychotic disorders hospitalizations associated with cannabis abuse or dependence: a nationwide big data analysis. Int J Methods Psychiatr Res. 2019;5:e1813.
24. Hasan A, von Keller R, Friemel C, Hall W, Schneider M, Koethe D, et al. Cannabis use and psychosis: a review of reviews. Eur Arch Psychiatry Clin Neurosci. 2019; https://doi.org/10.1007/s00406-019-01068-z.
25. Farrell M, Martin N, Stockings E, Bórquez A, Cepeda J, Degenhardt L, Ali R, Tran L, Rehm J, Torrens M, Shoptaw S, McKetin R. Responding to global stimulant use: challenges and opportunities. Lancet. 2019;394(10209):1652–67.
26. McKetin R, Leung J, Stockings E, Huo Y, Foulds J, Lappin J, Cumming C, Arunogiri S, Young J, Sara G, Farrell M, Degenhardt L. Mental health outcomes associated with of the use of amphetamines: a systematic review and meta-analysis. E Clin Med. 2019;17(16):81–97.
27. Gan H, Zhao Y, Jiang H, Zhu Y, Chen T, Tan H, Zhong N, Du J, Zhao M. A research of methamphetamine induced psychosis in 1,430 individuals with methamphetamine use disorder: clinical features and possible risk factors. Front Psych. 2018;6(9):551.
28. Moran L, Ongur D, Hsu J, Castro V, Perlis R, Schneeweiss S. Psychosis with methylphenidate or amphetamine in patients with ADHD. N Engl J Med. 2019;380(12):1128–38.
29. Otete H, Fleming M, West J, Orton E. Healthcare utilisation, morbidities and alcohol use monitoring prior to alcoholic psychosis diagnosis. Alcohol Alcohol. 2019;54(2):131–8.
30. Engelhard C, Touquet G, Tansens A, De Fruyt J. Psychotische stoornis door alcohol: een systematisch literatuuroverzicht. Tijdschr Psychiatr. 2015;57(3):192–201.
31. Kendler KS, Ohlsson H, Sundquist J, Sundquist K. Prediction of onset of substance-induced psychotic disorder and its progression to schizophrenia in a swedish national sample. Am. J. Psychiatry. 2019;176(9):711–9. https://doi.org/10.1176/appi.ajp.2019.18101217.
32. Mustonen A, Ahokas T, Nordström T, Murray G, Mäki P, Jääskeläinen E, Heiskala A, Mcgrath J, Scott J, Miettunen J, Niemelä S. Smokin' hot: adolescent smoking and the risk of psychosis. Acta Psychiatr Scand. 2018;138(1):5–14.
33. Lê Cook B, Wayne G, Nilay Kafali E, Liu Z, Shu C, Flores M. Trends in smoking among adults with mental illness and association between mental health treatment and smoking cessation. JAMA. 2014;311(2):172–82.

34. Hickling L, Perez-Iglesias R, Ortiz-García de la Foz V, Balanzá-Martínez V, McGuire P, Crespo-Facorro B, Ayesa-Arriola R. Tobacco smoking and its association with cognition in first episode psychosis patients. Schizophr Res. 2018 Feb;192:269–73.
35. Vermeulen J, Schirmbeck F, Blankers M, van Tricht M, van den Brink W, de Haan L. Genetic risk and outcome of psychosis (GROUP) investigators. Smoking, symptoms, and quality of life in patients with psychosis, siblings, and healthy controls: a prospective, longitudinal cohort study. Lancet. Psychiatry. 2019;6(1):25–34.
36. Gurillo P, Jauhar S, Murray R, MacCabe J. Does tobacco use cause psychosis? Systematic review and meta-analysis. Lancet Psychiatry. 2015;2:718–25.
37. Hunter A, Murray R, Asher L, Leonardi-Bee J. The effects of tobacco smoking, and prenatal tobacco smoke exposure, on risk of schizophrenia: a systematic review and meta-analysis. Nicotine Tob Res. 2018;22(1):3–10.
38. Scott J, Matuschka L, Niemelä S, Miettunen J, Emmerson B, Mustonen A. Evidence of a causal relationship between smoking tobacco and schizophrenia Spectrum disorders. Front Psych. 2018;20(9):607.
39. Awad A, Voruganti L. Revisiting the 'self-medication' hypothesis in light of the new data linking low striatal dopamine to comorbid addictive behavior. Ther Adv Psychopharmacol. 2015 Jun;5(3):172–8.
40. Varese F, Smeets F, Drukker M, Lieverse R, Lataster T, Viechtbauer W, Read J, van Os J, Bentall R. Childhood adversities increase the risk of psychosis: a meta-analysis of patient-control, prospective- and cross-sectional cohort studies. Schizophr Bull. 2012;38(4):661–71.
41. Turner S, Harvey C, Hayes L, Castle D, Galletly C, Sweeney S, Shah S, Keogh L, Spittal M. Childhood adversity and clinical and psychosocial outcomes in psychosis. Epidemiol Psychiatr Sci. 2019;16(29):e78.
42. Khokhar J, Dwiel L, Henricks A, Doucette W, Green A. The link between schizophrenia and substance use disorder: a unifying hypothesis. Schizophr Res. 2018;194:78–85. https://doi.org/10.1016/j.schres.2017.04.016.
43. Green A, Khokhar J. Addiction and schizophrenia: a translational perspective. Schizophr Res. 2018;194:1–3. https://doi.org/10.1016/j.schres.2017.10.008.
44. Read J, Bentall R, Dillon J, editors. Models of madness: psychological, social and biological approaches to psychosis. 2nd ed. London: Routledge; 2013.
45. Krause M, Huhn M, Schneider-Thoma J, Bighelli I, Gutsmiedl K, Leucht S. Efficacy, acceptability and tolerability of antipsychotics in patients with schizophrenia and comorbid substance use. A systematic review and meta-analysis. Eur Neuropsychopharmacol. 2019 Jan;29(1):32–45.
46. Lambert M, Conus P, Eide P, Mass R, Karow A, Moritz S, Golks D, Naber D. Impact of present and past antipsychotic side effects on attitude toward typical antipsychotic treatment and adherence. Eur Psychiatry. 2004;19(7):415–22.
47. Clerici M, de Bartolomeis A, De Filippis S, Ducci G, Maremmani I, Martinotti G, Schifano F. Patterns of Management of Patients with Dual Disorder (psychosis) in Italy: a survey of psychiatrists and other physicians focusing on clinical practice. Front Psych. 2018 Nov;13(9):575. https://doi.org/10.3389/fpsyt.2018.00575.
48. Archibald L, Brunette MF, Wallin DJ, Green AI. Alcohol use disorder and schizophrenia or schizoaffective disorder. Alcohol Res. 2019;40(1) https://doi.org/10.35946/arcr.v40.1.06.
49. Lev-Ran S, Balchand K, Lefebvre L, Araki KF, Le Foll B. Pharmacotherapy of alcohol use disorders and concurrent psychiatric disorders: a review. Can J Psychiatr. 2012;57(6):342–9. https://doi.org/10.1177/070674371205700603.
50. Das N, Mahapatra A, Sarkar S. Disulfiram induced psychosis: revisiting an age-old entity. Asian J Psychiatr. 2017;30:94–5. https://doi.org/10.1016/j.ajp.2017.08.011.
51. Mueser KT, Noordsy DL, Fox L, Wolfe R. Disulfiram treatment for alcoholism in severe mental illness. Am J Addict. 2003;12(3):242–52.
52. RCP. Royal College of Physicians, Royal College of Psychiatrists. In: Smoking and mental health. London; 2013. Royal College of Psychiatrists Council Report CR178.

53. Evins, AE, Benowitz, NL, West, R, Russ, C, McRae, T, Lawrence, D, . . . Anthenelli, RM. Neuropsychiatric safety and efficacy of Varenicline, bupropion, and nicotine patch in smokers with psychotic, anxiety, and mood disorders in the EAGLES trial. J Clin Psychopharmacol 2019. 39(2), 108–116. doi:https://doi.org/10.1097/JCP.0000000000001015.
54. Peckham E, Brabyn S, Cook L, Tew G, Gilbody S. Smoking cessation in severe mental ill health: what works? An updated systematic review and meta-analysis. BMC Psychiatry. 2017;17(1):252.
55. Valentine GW, Hefner K, Jatlow PI, Rosenheck RA, Gueorguieva R, Sofuoglu M. Impact of E-cigarettes on smoking and related outcomes in veteran smokers with psychiatric comorbidity. J Dual Diagn. 2018;14(1):2–13. https://doi.org/10.1080/15504263.2017.1384877.
56. Kern AM, Akerman SC, Nordstrom BR. Opiate dependence in schizophrenia: case presentation and literature review. J Dual Diagn. 2014;10(1):52–7. https://doi.org/10.1080/15504263.2013.867199.

4 Recovery from Psychosis: Definition, Paradoxes, and Clinical Implications

Paul H. Lysaker

4.1 Introduction

In the 1960s and 1970s, it was accepted that people diagnosed with psychosis would have a course of progressive decline. They were expected to be unable to ever return to work, form romantic bonds, or function as full members within their communities. At best it was accepted that with prolonged pharmacological treatment they might become "stable," which is to say not endure any more substantial losses. This view has been challenged in the time since and a significantly different account has emerged [1]. Contrary to these assertions which had been previously accepted as fact, broadly based research has confirmed that people with psychosis do not experience a process of continuous decline which ends in dysfunction and chronic disability. Instead, people who have been diagnosed with psychosis can be said to recover in ways that are consequential and measurable, no matter the severity of the disorder they had previously experienced. This work suggests an optimistic view in which there is reason to believe that regardless of how ill, disordered, or disorganized a person might have been during a period characterized as acute psychosis, the possibilities which make for a meaningful life remain available to them in the future.

The recognition of the inaccuracy of pessimistic views of outcome in psychosis have attracted much support and led to the reforms across multiple domains of allied fields of mental health. Among other things, it has iteratively spurred the development of models of wellness and the requirements of treatment that promote wellness, provoking new questions, and advances in both theory and application. For example, awareness that health should be an expected outcome, rather than stability and decline has raised the issue of what health should look like beyond

P. H. Lysaker (✉)
Roudebush Veteran Affairs Medical Center, Indianapolis, IN, USA

Department of Psychiatry, Indiana University School of Medicine, Indianapolis, IN, USA
e-mail: plysaker@iupui.edu

P. Rocca, S. Bellino (eds.), *Psychosis and Personality Disorders*,
https://doi.org/10.1007/978-3-031-09058-5_4

being the absence of negative outcomes and in particular viewed from whose perspective? This changing view of outcome has also offered new opportunities to think about what the key ingredients of a clinical intervention are which should be expected to promote these outcomes. It has also challenged existing treatments which may inadvertently offer barriers to these kinds of outcomes.

To explore these issues, this chapter will first critically examine earlier pessimistic views of outcomes in psychosis. We will then discuss the emergence of the concept of recovery and the research efforts it has spurred on. We will focus here on what we propose to be two key issues which this research has raised, and which have yet to be resolved: how to understand recovery as a matter both of the perspective of the people who have been given the diagnosis and of the perspective of others, and how to locate the ultimate health-related outcomes in terms of community membership. Following this, we will discuss the potential of research on metacognition in psychosis to offer possible solutions to these issues and examine possible ways to respond to these issues. Finally, we will explore the clinical implications of work on metacognition for recovery-oriented treatments in light of these issues.

4.2 Historical Views of Outcome from Psychosis: The Rule and Alure of Pessimism

Historically pessimistic views of outcomes from psychosis have multiple roots, though they are most often associated with the work of Kraepelin [2]. Kraepelin, on the basis of interviews with people with long histories of institutionalized care without subsequent improvement, proposed that there exists a disease defined by its unremitting course ending in severe dysfunction: dementia praecox or precocious dementia. He firmly assumed this must reflect the gradual decline of brain function which ultimately resulted in a mental state he described phenomenologically and metaphorically as an orchestra which had no conductor or organizing function.

For many potentially different reasons, Kraepelin's view of a precocious dementia was embraced by many. For one, in essence this view allowed for ubiquitous treatment failures by virtue of positing a process that could not be addressed by care. This view held that the declines so broadly observed among people living in institutional settings were the result of aberrant processes, potentially suggested in some portions of this work to be metabolic in nature for which no current treatments were available [3]. Institutions and practitioners were thus absolved from any responsibility for treatment failure. Further, with a new apparently scientific label there was not the potential, albeit possibility in the distant future of a cure, and so while treatment failure in the moment was inevitable there was no reason to hold out hope for the future, but also no immediate need for a change in those institutions themselves.

Thus, one of the major attractions for the work of Kraepelin may have been its neglect and diversion from the obvious possibility that the terrible outcomes noted in psychiatric institutions were the direction result of inhumane and unethical conditions found in those institutions. For example, the progressive decline might well be expected in intuitions where instead of hospitable care, people were subjected to interventions involuntarily imposed which were likely harmful. Such procedures presented as treatments included emetics and exposure to simulated drowning [4, 5].

While there was considerable acceptance of Kraepelin's views, others and in particular Bleuler [6], offered a more nuanced account of psychosis, one that went beyond its surface features and sought to describe the experience of the person who had been diagnosed. Bleuler, in contrast to Kraepelin, was reported to have spent time getting to know his patients and therefore did more than observe their oddities and inconsistencies. He also had an interest in emerging views within psychiatry of the complexity of the alterations in consciousness that occurred in psychosis including those of Freud [7]. Bleuler thus turned explicitly away from the odd and inexplicable behaviors of patients and focused on three aspects of the experience a person in the world which he believed were disturbed or rendered fragmentary in psychosis. He proposed to discard the term dementia praecox in favor of "schizophrenia," a term which meant the fragmentation of thought, affect and desire. He observed roughly the same levels of dysfunction among his patients as Kraepelin, but instead of a progressive dementia he said this kind of dysfunction, which he labeled as autism, was a result of the fragmentation of experience [8].

While Bleuler suggested that these alterations in the experience of thought, affect, and desire were likely the result of aberrant biological processes, he allowed that they could be the subject of treatment, allowing space for recovery where previously there had been none. If, for example, a person could find a way to overcome their experience of the fragmentation of their thoughts, emotions, and wishes, they might find a way to make their way in life again.

This thread though seemed to be quickly lost. In place of a person who found the world incomprehensible, views emerged of people with psychosis which emphasized the oddness of their thinking and even the lack of pain and distress, something referred to as non-affective psychosis. The disorder was cast as a matter of inexplicable experience [9]. The consequence of this was for many decades after these original assertions, the allied fields of mental health held onto the deeply pessimistic views of outcome noted in the introduction of this paper. Incomprehensive experiences led to incomprehensible and irreversible dysfunction with no mechanism by which processes that culminated in recovery could even begin to coalesce.

4.3 The Emergence of Recovery as the Expected Outcome from Psychosis

It is not clear exactly how these pessimistic views came to begin to fade, but one tipping point seems likely to be tied to the emergence of opportunities for people who had been diagnosed with psychosis to share their experience of acute psychosis and what followed those acute periods [10]. Whereas previous research had considered outcome to be a matter best described by expert observers of psychosis, new work turned to the experience of people who live with these conditions. This work included longitudinal research wherein people diagnosed with psychosis much earlier in their lives in both Europe and North America were interviewed, revealing that many, if not most, had found ways to have satisfying lives [e.g., 11, 12]. In parallel, a growing grassroots movement began to challenge barriers placed by the psychiatric community to the possibility that people diagnosed with psychosis could achieve a genuinely acceptable and fully meaningful quality of life. This work also relied on the experience of people diagnosed with psychosis.

This work, regardless of its methodology, then began to coalesce around a series of findings that shared common themes. Recovery from psychosis was possible and not uncommon [13]. Considering measurable behaviors including attaining vocational and social outcomes as well as symptom remission, this work as summarized by Leonhardt et al. [14], found rates of symptom remission in adults diagnosed with early psychosis ranged from over one in three to nine in ten, with both short- and long-term follow up periods. The reattainment of adequate psychosocial function in this same group ranged from three in ten to more than one in two with 14%–30% achieving both good psychosocial and symptom outcomes. A similar pattern, though slightly more positive, was also found in studies of prolonged psychosis.

Other studies have focused more directly on a person's own experiences of themselves following a diagnosis of psychosis. One approach to this has involved objective self-assessment using the Recovery Assessment Scale (RAS) [15]. This instrument provides a summary quantitative estimate of a person's experience of recovery including their degree of hope, goal orientation, willingness to ask for help, sense of connection to others, and not feeling overwhelmed by symptoms. Research has found links between these reports and objective ratings of emotional distress and sense of community involvement [16, 17]. Using qualitative methods, other studies have sought to more carefully uncover how recovery is experienced by recovering people as fundamentally related to sense of self [18]. In a synthesis of qualitative studies, McCarthy-Jones et al. [19] found that recovery involved the reversal of alterations in sense of self, purpose, and connection to others that commonly accompanied psychosis, while Soundy et al. [20] found that the subjective experience of recovery required an adjustment to the experience of psychosis, self-management, and social support. One prominent framework, referred to as CHIME, suggests that for people diagnosed with psychosis to recover there needs to be the emergence connectedness to others, hope, identity, meaning in life, and a sense of personal agency [21]. Ellison et al. [22], exploring recent reviews, found that for people to experience themselves as recovering, they needed to make gains in identity, empowerment, meaning in life, and hopefulness.

Pessimistic views of outcome reduced any pressure on the development of recovery-oriented interventions. In contrast, the research noted above has had the opposite effect, accelerating work on intervention. Though recovery remained ignored in some mainstream diagnostic manuals [23], influential guidelines were proposed from groups that included people who had been diagnosed with psychosis which placed recovery as the desired outcome of treatment [24]. Across varying mental health settings, clinical services were identified as needing to move beyond the promotion of stability to the identification and dismantling of barriers to recovery. Services, for example, emerged which were increasingly concerned with community inclusion [25], the rejection of internalized stigma [26], and the recognition of the concept of recovery [27]. Even the names of programs were commonly changed to reflect an emphasis on recovery [28].

4.4 Two Emerging Challenges or Paradoxes from Research on Recovery from Psychosis

While the work summarized so far overturned long standing views of outcome, it has also raised a number of challenges or paradoxes. For the purposes of this chapter, we will focus on two related ones. First, recovery, as it has been studied, may vary according to who is evaluating it: the person with a diagnosis of psychosis or someone else. As has been noted elsewhere [29], some of the important experiences that people diagnosed with psychosis may have as they recover are fundamentally subjective and not observable by others. Further, the criteria others may use to define recovery, namely the remission of defining features of psychosis, may be of less importance to diagnosed people. Thus, people may experience themselves as fully in recovery and not be regarded as recovered by others. In parallel, diagnosed people may not feel they have made significant progress toward recovery while others believe they have. As an illustration, a diagnosed person may feel they have recaptured a fully meaningful sense of self and hope and connections to others and feel they have recovered, while family members, noticing symptoms or a lack of work, conclude that recovery has not occurred. As an example of the mirror image of this dilemma, a clinician may note symptom remission and independent housing as signs of recovery, but the person still without a firm sense of identity and agency may feel far from meaningfully recovered. Research that bears out this paradox includes recent studies suggesting many who experience themselves as recovered are not necessarily identified as such by objective measures [30], as well as other work suggesting that the meaning of objective outcomes can only be fully understood in the context of subjective experiences that can be revealed in qualitative methods [31].

A second related, though more abstract paradox concerns *where* recovery takes place as opposed to how it should be defined. Again, focusing on the perspective of the person making a judgement about recovery, we find that people diagnosed with psychosis experience their recovery as occurring within their communities. They feel they have recovered because they again belong somewhere and can locate themselves as being members of their community [14]. Put yet another way, they recover in the world through connections to a larger group. This view of recovery as occurring in the community may then be contrasted with an alternative view in which changes within the brain or individual are touted as the fundamental site of recovery [32]. This may even be seen to create strange bedfellows that include recovery as occurring at a biological substrate and other views of recovery as something only one person can achieve with little say so from the larger world. In either case, the place where recovery occurs would seem to again be within the person.

Of note, there are potentially simple solutions. For example, some writers distinguish personal recovery from clinical recovery [33]. Others allow for a range of different outcomes which can occur at different locations. Thus, some kinds of recovery are observable by others and some by the recovering person while some kinds of recovery occur in the community and some within the person. The issue we have with this explanation is that it may fragment the concept of recovery and allows it to begin to mean so many things as to have no agreeable conceptual basis. It allows for people to both be recovered and not recovered across a range of different locations. Certainly, this also poses a barrier to comprehensive services which seek a holistic view of the person as living in their community. For example, how should we understand the dilemmas of the diagnosed person and others having different ideas about whether recovery has occurred? Supporting the possibility that there can be deeper connections underneath these paradoxes is research suggesting a complex, yet unclear relationship among recovery as assessed from different views [16, 34–36].

4.5 Metacognition and Paradoxes Posed by the Study of Recovery

One common denominator across the paradoxes of what defines recovery and where it takes place involves people making decisions about what has gone wrong and interrupted the life of a diagnosed person and what would constitute a return to health. Thus, meaning has to be made of both disorder and health.

One branch of research which has been directly concerned with meaning making and also understanding what core processes may underlie psychosis has focused on the construct of metacognition [29]. This work understands metacognition using an integrative framework as a far-reaching set of processes that allow people to notice and reflect upon experience at many levels including cognitive, emotional, and embodied aspects [37]. Metacognitive capacity thus allows people to perceive and think about different pieces of experience, both on their own and in terms of their relationship to one another [38, 39]. When functioning efficiently, metacognitive capacities allow awareness of specific thoughts, feelings and bodily states and to see how they fit into a larger sense of oneself and one's connection to the world [29]. They allow for people to have available to themselves within the flow of life a sense of how to respond to the questions of who am I, what is happening, and what should I do about it. They also make available an idea of deeper questions as well as what is the larger purpose of one's life and what is the nature of one's connection to others [40]. Applied to psychosis, this research has suggested that metacognitive deficits or reductions in metacognitive capacity could leave people with a relatively more fragmented sense of the self, one which may have a limited sense of purpose and position within their community. Considering recovery, metacognitive deficits may complicate a person's ability to make cohesive and coherent sense of what has happened to them that could be associated with a diagnosis of psychosis and what they want to do about that. It would thus be difficult to know how to achieve some of the most subjective, as well as objective markers to recovery. Evidence supporting this includes findings of greater deficits in metacognitive capacity within the personal narratives among people diagnosed with psychosis compared to people diagnosed with other forms of mental illness often considered less severe than psychosis, and community members without any diagnosis of mental illness. A lesser degree of metacognitive deficits among people diagnosed with psychosis have also been associated with greater levels of objective and subjective degrees of wellness [29]. Similarly, the improvement in metacognition with targeted intervention have been found to be associated with improvements in both objective and subjective indicators of wellness [41].

Turning back to the issue of how to think about recovery and the differences that can be found between a diagnosed person's sense or recovery versus the view of another, we suggest that metacognition may offer an objective measurement of the processes that support how well a recovering person is making sense of their challenges and deciding how to manage them. This view allows that people will have different views of whether recovery is occurring, but because at the core the matter of recovery is about a diagnosed person making a kind of sense that others can understand of what has happened to them and what they want and need, disagreements can be partially resolved.

As an illustration consider the earlier example of a recovering person who felt they had recovered while others had not. Here the issue would come down to whether the recovering person had made coherent sense of the challenges and possibilities they faced and how they wanted to proceed. This would allow for recovery to include any number of ways in which a person might validly disagree with others. For example, a person might coherently understand what happened to them in the course of psychosis as related to a history of abuse and hence how recovering some degree of self-compassion represented the deepest form of recovery, regardless of whether they continued to not work and held beliefs others considered idiosyncratic. This is not to say that recovery could be anything. The meanings made of the challenges and possibilities within a life interrupted by a diagnosis of psychosis have to be accessible to others. As a further example, understanding the challenges of mental illness as the result of forces that are at odds with virtually everyone else's beliefs in the community, for example, the belief one is God, would not be judged as part of recovery. Nor would acts not sanctioned as healthy within one's community, such as committing crimes. As a final example, the same process could be observed for the person who denies they have recovered. Again, the issue would rest on the coherence of the person's understanding of their challenges. For example, having achieved things that others value could naturally not be understood as part of recovery if the diagnosed person does not share those values.

Turning to the issue of where recovery occurs, the metacognitive model provides another bridge, though a more complex one. Metacognition in the model described above involves not only consideration of many aspects of experience (e.g., cognitive, emotional, and embodied) but is also a fundamentally intersubjective process [42]. In parallel with the observations made above, meanings made of the challenges and possibilities for a life interrupted by a diagnosis of psychosis have to be made with others, either in direct dialogue with those others or in ways that allow for potential dialogue. In this sense, recovery actually cannot just take place in the mind of the recovering person or the others who are thinking about their recovery, rather it has to take place jointly between the diagnosed person and others in their larger communities. Following the observation of William James [50], no one has a direct sense of self. We know ourselves as we experience the world. Accordingly, recovery is also taking place in the world in the larger sense of people are beings in the world always in relation to one another.

4.6 General Implications for Recovery-Oriented Practice and Conclusions

In summary, we have suggested that with the understanding that recovery is an obtainable outcome from psychosis optimism has arisen but so have several paradoxes. Those include the problems that recovery may depend upon who is observing it and that it is unclear where recovery might be said to occur exactly. As a partial solution to these paradoxes, we have presented research on metacognition in psychosis which may allow us to see that the experience of recovery, regardless of who is observing it or where it occurs, is a matter of an attempt to make coherent meaning of the challenges and possibilities within a life interrupted by a diagnosis of psychosis and hence differences in perspective are to be expected and can be resolved. This view also helps place recovery as a process that is always happening between people within their communities.

We would suggest that this view, while not offering a complete resolution of these issues, allows recovery to be understood as a holistic process and accordingly has several immediate clinical implications. For the purposes of concluding this chapter we will suggest four. First, without regard to the content or theoretical basis for a specific treatment or intervention, to promote recovery it must involve a dialogue in which there is a joint examination of the possibilities and dilemmas facing that person. That dialogue has to be respectful, with both parties having the possibility of having their own unique insight.

Second, this dialogue may be challenging for both parties as both face the uncertainty that comes with joint meaning making in the face of pain. As in most complicated human affairs, there will rarely be only one right decision. This is to say this dialogue will not be value free and may ultimately be about risk and not the simple amelioration of pain. This risk is further one that is shared [43]. For example, deciding to reduce or discontinue antipsychotic medication may risk rehospitalization, while deciding to date or work may risk rejection and confirm negative thoughts about the self. As diagnosed people come to think differently about themselves, they may also lose previous systems of meaning [44]. Deciding which risks to take then seems to be required of any treatment which will promote recovery and making that decision would naturally seem to involve reflection upon the meanings that different risks and possibilities have for the diagnosed person. This, from an intersubjective framework would seem to require the sharing of not just thoughts about concrete realities but the sharing of both very real anxieties and hope.

Third, these kinds of interventions, therefore, require ongoing negotiation about the working alliance and the role of the clinician and recovering person within it [40]. The focus of the intervention and the goals have to be continuously re-evaluated as well as the kind of role the treater is expected to and willing to fulfill.

The fourth clinical implication we would like to draw attention to is the assessment of the metacognitive capacity of the person diagnosed with psychosis. If as suggested by work on metacognition, making sense of challenges and possibilities is fundamentally a metacognitive act, then the dialogue within treatment about these issues may also need to be sensitive to the recovering person's current capacity for metacognition. Indeed arriving at a shared understanding with people diagnosed with psychosis rests on the formation of ideas whose complexity does not exceed either person's metacognitive capacity. Thus, treaters may have the onus of assessing the metacognitive capacity of the person diagnosed with psychosis on a relatively continuous basis and accordingly adjusting the complexity of the ideas they are seeking to jointly form. One tool that has been used for this purpose in psychotherapy is the Metacognition Assessment Scale-Abbreviated [29, 41, 45], though it is likely other approaches could be used.

Of note, there are limitations important to consider. First long-term longitudinal research is needed that examines the perceptions of recovery between people diagnosed with psychosis and others including treaters, family, and community members. Such work may parse out the different features of recovery and suggest new solutions to the paradoxes noted here. The measurement of metacognition is also in its infancy and most studies have involved people enrolled in treatment. Work is needed to develop more fine-grained means of assessment and more diverse samples. Concerning practice, we have suggested overall processes, but research is needed to explore how these are best incorporated into practice across different settings and with different kinds of providers. Work is needed to explore elements of recovery that indeed may affect outcome more than others.

References

1. Hamm JA, Rutherford E, Wiesepape CN, Lysaker PH. Community mental health practice in the United States: past, present, and future. Consortium Psychiatricum. 2020;1:7–13.
2. Kraepelin E, Barclay RM, Robertson GM. Dementia praecox and Paraphrenia. Edinburgh: E&S Livingstone; 1919.
3. Noll R. American madness: the rise and fall of dementia praecox. Cambridge, MA: Harvard University Press; 2011.
4. Hinshaw S. Another kind of madness. New York, NY: St Martin's Press; 2017.
5. Whitaker R. Mad in America: bad science, bad medicine, and the enduring mistreatment of the mentally ill. New York, NY: Perseus Publishing; 2002.
6. Bleuler E. Dementia praecox or the Group of Schizophrenias. Zinkin J, trans. New York, NY: International Universities; 1950. Original work published 1911
7. Freud S. On narcissism: an introduction. Standard Edition. 1914;14:67–102.

8. Katschnig H. Psychiatry's contribution to the public stereotype of schizophrenia: historical considerations. J Eval Clin Pract. 2018;24(5):1093–100.
9. Jaspers K. General psychopathology. New York, NY: John Hopkins Univeristy Press; 1997. *Original work published 1959*
10. Roe D. Recovering from severe mental illness: mutual influences of self and illness. J Psychosoc Nurs Ment Health Serv. 2005;43:35–40.
11. Ciompi L. The natural history of schizophrenia in the long term. Br J Psychiatry. 1980;136:413–20.
12. Harding CM, Brooks GW, Ashikaga T, Strauss JS, Breier A. The Vermont longitudinal study of persons with severe mental illness I: methodology, study sample, and overall status 32 years later. Am J Psychiatry. 1987;144(6):718–26.
13. Anthony WA. Recovery from mental illness: the guiding vision of the mental health service system in the 1990s. Psychosoc Rehabil J. 1993;16(4):11–23.
14. Leonhardt BL, Huling K, Hamm JA, Roe D, Hasson-Ohayon I, McLeod H, et al. Recovery and serious mental illness: A review of current clinical and research paradigms and future directions. Expert Rev Neurother. 2017;17(11):1117–30.
15. Corrigan PW, Giffort D, Rashid F, Leary M, Okeke I. Recovery as a psychological construct. Community Ment Health J. 1999;35(3):231–9.
16. Jorgensen R, Zoffmann V, Munk-Jorgensen P, Buck KD, Jensen SO, Hasson I, et al. Relationships over time of subjective and objective elements of recovery in persons with schizophrenia. Psychiatry Res. 2015;228(1):14–9.
17. Garverich S, Prener CG, Guyer ME, Lincoln AK. What matters: factors impacting the recovery process among outpatient mental health service users. Psychiatr Rehabil J. 2020; https://doi.org/10.1037/prj0000407.
18. Andresen R, Caputi P, Oades L. Stages of recovery instrument: development of a measure of recovery from serious mental illness. Aust N Z J Psychiatry. 2006;40(11–12):972–80.
19. McCarthy-Jones S, Marriott M, Knowles R, Rowse G, Thompson AR. What is psychosis? A meta-synthesis of inductive qualitative studies exploring the experience of psychosis. Psychosis. 2013;5(1):1–16.
20. Soundy A, Stubbs B, Roskell C, Williams SE, Fox A, Vancampfort D. Identifying the facilitators and processes which influence recovery in individuals with schizophrenia: a systematic review and thematic synthesis. J Ment Health. 2015;24(2):103–10.
21. Leamy M, Bird V, Le Boutilier C, Williams J, Slade L. Conceptual framework for personal recovery in mental health: systematic review and narrative synthesis. Br J Psychiatry. 2011;199(6):445–52.
22. Ellison ML, Belanger LK, Niles BL, Evans LC, Bauer MS. Explication and definition of mental health recover: A systematic review. Admin Pol Ment Health. 2018;45(1):91–102.
23. Nemeroff CB, Weinberger D, Rutter M, Macmillan HL, Bryant RA, Wessely S, Stein DJ, Pariante CM, Seemüller F, Berk M, Malhi GS, Preisig M, Brüne M, Lysaker PH. DSM-5: A collection of psychiatrist views on the changes, controversies, and future directions. BMC Med. 2013;11:202.
24. Substance Abuse and Mental Health Services Administration (SAMHSA). SAMHSA's working definition of recovery [Internet]. 2012. Available from: https://store.samhsa.gov/sites/default/files/d7/priv/pep12-recdef.pdf
25. Tanaka K, Davidson L, Craig TJ. Sense of clubhouse community belonging and empowerment. Int J Soc Psychiatry. 2018;64(3):276–85.
26. Yanos PT, Roe D, Lysaker PH. The impact of illness identity on recovery from severe mental illness. Am J Psychiatr Rehabil. 2010;13(2):73–93.
27. McGuire AB, Bartholomew T, Anderson AI, Bauer SM, McGrew JH, White DA, Luther L, Rollins A, Pereira A, Salyers MP. Illness management and recovery in community practice. Psychiatr Rehabil J. 2016;39(4):343–51. https://doi.org/10.1037/prj0000200. Epub 2016 Aug 8. PMID: 27505349; PMCID: PMC5125841.]
28. Nelson CB, Bowersox N, King J, Hunt MG. Psychometric examination of care quality measures in VA psychosocial rehabilitation and recovery centers (PRRCs). Psychol Serv. 2020;17(3):300–10. https://doi.org/10.1037/ser0000357. Epub 2019 May 23. PMID: 31120292

29. Lysaker PH, Kukla M, Leonhardt BL, Hamm JA, Schnackenberg Martin A, Zalzala AB, Gagen EC, Hasson-Ohayon I. Meaning, integration, and the self in serious mental illness: Implications of research in metacognition for psychiatric rehabilitation. J Psychiatr Rehabil. 2020; https://doi.org/10.1037/prj0000436.
30. Boggian I, Lamonaca D, Ghisi M, Bottesi G, Svettini A, Basso L, Bernardelli K, Merlin S, Liberman RP, S.I.R. 2 group. "The Italian Study on Recovery 2" Phase 1: Psychometric Properties of the Recovery Assessment Scale (RAS), Italian Validation of the Recovery Assessment Scale. Front Psychiatry. 2020;10:1000. https://doi.org/10.3389/fpsyt.2019.01000. PMID: 32119004; PMCID: PMC7013090
31. Hasson-Ohayon I, Roe D, Yanos PT, Lysaker PH. The trees and the forest: mixed methods in the assessment of psychosocial interventions' processes and outcomes in psychiatry. J Ment Health. 2015;26(6):543–9.
32. Nasrallah HA. We are physicians, not providers and we treat patients, not clients! Curr Psychiatr Ther. 2020;19(2):5–7,29.
33. Lim MW, Remington G, Lee J. Personal recovery in serious mental illness: making sense of the concept. Ann Acad Med Singap. 2017;46(1):29–31.
34. Thomas EC, Muralidharan A, Medoff D, Drapalski AL. Self-efficacy as a mediator of the relationship between social support and recovery in serious mental illness. Psychiatr Rehabil J. 2016;39(4):352–60.
35. Shadmi E, Gelkopf M, Garber-Epstein P, Baloush-Kleinman V, Doudai R, Roe D. Routine patient reported outcomes as predictors of psychiatric rehospitalization. Schizophr Res. 2017;192:119–23.
36. Kukla M, Lysaker PH, Roe D. Strong subjective recovery as a protective factor against the effects of positive symptoms on quality of life outcomes in schizophrenia. Compr Psychiatry. 2014;55(6):1363–8.
37. Moritz S, Lysaker PH. Metacognition–what did James H. Flavell really say and the implications for the conceptualization and design of metacognitive interventions. Schizophr Res. 2018;201:20–6.
38. Lysaker PH, Dimaggio G. Metacognitive capacities for reflection in schizophrenia: implications for developing treatments. Schizophr Bull. 2014;40(3):487–91.
39. Lysaker PH, Keane J, Poirier-Culleton S, Lundin N. Schizophrenia, recovery and the self: an introduction to the special issue on metacognition. Schizophr Res Cogn. 2020;19:100167.
40. Lysaker PH, Lysaker JT. Disturbances in dialogue and metacognition: A renewed way to understand and respond to alterations in self-experience in psychosis. Theory Psychol. 2020; https://doi.org/10.1177/0959354320973752.
41. Lysaker PH, Gagen EC, Klion R, Zalzala AB, Vohs J, Faith LA, et al. Metacognitive reflection and insight therapy: A recovery-oriented treatment approach for psychosis. Psychol Res Behav Manag. 2020;13:331–41.
42. Hasson-Ohayon I, Gumley A, McLeod H, Lysaker PH. Metacognition and intersubjectivity: Reconsidering their relationship following advances from the study of persons with psychosis. Frontiers. 11:567. https://doi.org/10.3389/fpsyg.2020.00567. eCollection 2020
43. Zisman-Ilani Y, Lysaker PH, Hasson-Ohayon I. Shard risk-taking: shared decision making in serious mental illness. Psychiatr Serv. 2020;72(4):461–3.
44. Buck KD, Roe D, Yanos PT, Buck B, Fogely R, Grant M, et al. Challenges to assisting with the recovery of personal identity and wellness for persons with serious mental illness: considerations for mental health professionals. Psychosis. 2013;5(2):134–43.
45. Lysaker PH, Klion R. Recovery, meaning making, and severe mental illness: A comprehensive guide to metacognitive and reflection insight therapy. New York, NY: Routledge; 2017.

Cluster A Personality Disorders and Potential for Early Intervention in Psychosis: Challenges and Opportunities

5

Saeed Farooq and Muhammad Ayub

5.1 Cluster A Personality Disorders (CAPD): Classification and Symptoms

The Diagnostic and Statistical Manual of Mental Disorders, Fifth Edition (DSM-V) [1] classifies personality disorders in three clusters. The personality disorders within a 'cluster' share a number of common features and therefore are grouped together. The 'Cluster A' personality disorders consist of paranoid, schizoid and schizotypal personality disorders. The common features of personality disorders in this cluster are; social awkwardness, social withdrawal, odd or eccentric behaviour and distorted thinking.

Paranoid Personality Disorder (PPD) is characterized by a pervasive distrust and suspiciousness of other people, and sometimes by displaying pathological jealousy traits. The distorted thinking in people with PPD manifests in perception of the environment, such as reading malevolent intentions into genuinely harmless, innocuous comments or behaviour.

Schizoid Personality Disorder (SPD) is characterized by a pervasive pattern of social detachment, a restricted range of emotional expression and being socially isolated. Those with SPD do not seem to seek out or enjoy close relationships. People suffering SPD seem aloof, detached and mostly pursue solitary activities. They may be oblivious to social nuances and cues. Therefore, they appear to be socially inept and superficial. SPD is distinguished from paranoid and schizotypal PD by the prominence of social, interpersonal and affective deficits which sometimes resemble the negative symptoms of schizophrenia.

S. Farooq (✉)
School of Medicine, Keele University, Keele, UK

Midlands Partnership NHS Foundation Trust, Stafford, UK
e-mail: s.farooq@keele.ac.uk

M. Ayub
University College London, London, England, United Kingdom

P. Rocca, S. Bellino (eds.), *Psychosis and Personality Disorders*,
https://doi.org/10.1007/978-3-031-09058-5_5

Schizotypal Personality Disorder (SzPD) is characterized by an acute discomfort in social settings, and a reduced capacity for close relationships. People with SzPD tend to be socially isolated, reserved and distant. Unlike SPD, they also experience perceptual and cognitive distortions and/or eccentric behaviour. These perceptual abnormalities may include hallucination-like experiences. They may harbour odd beliefs, for instance, they may believe they can read other people's thoughts, or that their own thoughts are known to other people. These odd or superstitious beliefs and fantasies are inconsistent with cultural norms and may fluctuate with time in severity [1].

The International Classification of Mental and Behavioural Disorders, Tenth Edition (ICD-10) [2] does not use the cluster approach in classification of personality disorders. Contrary to the DSM approach, schizotypal disorder is classified as a psychosis-related disorder in ICD-10, as well as in the proposed ICD-11 [3]. The paranoid and schizoid personality disorders are classified under the disorders of personality and behaviour (F60-F69). The draft 11th edition of the International Classification of Diseases (ICD-11) adopts a dimensional approach to the classification of Personality Disorders that focuses on global levels of severity and five trait qualifiers [4]. Despite different approaches in classification, clinical features of these personality disorders are broadly similar in ICD-10 and DSM-V.

In the discussion below, we will refer to three personality disorders as specified in Cluster A of DSM-V. This is not due to better evidence for the validity of the Cluster A personality disorders in DSM-V, or any inherent strength of the cluster approach. We believe the clustering of these personality disorders is clinically useful, especially in the context of recent developments in concepts such as 'clinically high risk' states for psychosis and 'early intervention in psychosis'.

This chapter will focus mainly on the relationship of these disorders with schizophrenia and clinically high-risk states for psychosis. It will also focus on interventions for treating these disorders and their potential role in early psychosis treatment. The pathophysiology, aetiology, epidemiology and phenomenology will not be covered in detail here. The assessment tools, classification, treatment, history, epidemiology, heritability and genetics, cognitive impairments, social-affective disturbances and neurobiology of these disorders are reviewed in recent literature [5, 6], Similarly Barrantes-Vidal et al. [7] provide a good insight into the role of schizotypy in the aetiology of schizophrenia spectrum disorders [7]. There are also useful clinical reviews [8, 9].

Cluster A personality disorders, especially schizoid and schizotypal have a long history and are well described in phenomenological literature (see below). The prevalence of these disorders is higher than personality disorders that are commonly present in psychiatric practice, such as borderline personality disorder. Torgersen et al. [10] report population prevalence rates of 2.4% for paranoid personality disorder, 1.7% for schizoid personality disorder and 0.6% for schizotypal personality disorder. Similar prevalence rates were found in pooled data from ten community studies [10]. The prevalence of paranoid personality disorder indicates that it is among the most common personality disorders, with estimates suggesting a prevalence varying from 2.4% [10] to 4.41% [11].

Despite the relatively high prevalence, significant burden of disease and the relationship with severe mental illness, these personality disorders are less well studied in the modern literature and in clinical research. One reason may be that conditions such as Paranoid personality disorder, though chronic and disabling, are not commonly encountered in clinical settings as patients are generally very reluctant to seek treatment. It appears that the recent emergence of concepts such as 'At Risk Mental State' [12] that share a number of clinical features with these personality disorders have further shifted the focus away from these personality disorders.

5.2 Relationship between Cluster A Personality Disorders and Schizophrenia

Personality disorders are sometimes conceptualized as part of a spectrum with the axis I psychiatric disorders [13]. This argument has some face validity and is supported by the frequent associations (comorbidity) of each mental state disorder with its personality counterpart [14]. As we discuss below, this is particularly true for cluster A personality disorders.

Fonseca Pedrero and Debbané [15] suggested that schizophrenia, schizoaffective disorder, affective psychosis and psychotic disorder induced by substances, as well as schizoid, schizotypal and paranoid personality disorders belong to Psychotic-spectrum disorders. Phenomenologically, cluster A personality disorders have much in common with schizophrenia, with schizotypal personality disorder having strongest links with schizophrenia. These include a rich history related to schizotypy, phenomenological similarities and genetic, physiologic and neuroanatomical abnormalities that are common between schizophrenia and SzPD. The close relationship between schizotypal personality disorder and schizophrenia is reflected in its classification in ICD-10, as being part of psychosis.

The schizotypy and schizotypal personality disorders have their origin in the concepts of Bleuler's schizophrenia latens [16] which remained a conceptual guide for understanding phenotypic and clinical understandings of schizophrenia for many decades. Although Schizotypy is not recognized as such in modern classifications, it remains an interesting concept. This is shown by a recent spate of articles on its origins and relationship with schizophrenia [17–21]. Recently a supplement to Schizophrenia Bulletin was devoted to the conceptual and methodological issues related to schizotypy and provides useful guidance on the subject [22].

The term schizotypal personality disorder is a recent psychiatric nosological concept developed by Spitzer at the end of the 1970s and included in DSM [23]. The origins of schizotypal personality disorder can be traced to the beginning of the past century in a rich and long tradition of schizotypy. The term schizotypy refers to a latent personality structure that potentially has the liability for schizophrenia and can give rise to a variety of schizophrenia-related phenotypic outcomes [24]. Historically, the concept of schizotypy is not restricted to the clinical features that are associated with schizotypal personality disorders now a day. As discussed in detail by Lenzenweger, the 'schizotypic persons' may indeed display some of the phenomenology associated with schizotypal personality disorder, but they may also have other phenomenology which is not part of the SzPD as we know it today [20, 25].

It has been argued that SzPD represents an intermediate schizophrenia-spectrum phenotype, and therefore, can provide a better understanding of the genetics, pathogenesis, and treatment of related psychotic illnesses [6]. Both family and adoptive studies [26, 27] suggest a greater prevalence of schizotypal personality disorder in the relatives of patients with schizophrenia than in comparison groups. The prevalence of schizophrenia-related personality disorders and psychosis are higher in the relatives of schizophrenia probands than in the relatives of affective disorder probands [28, 29]. Similarly, patients with schizotypal personality disorder share a number of psychophysiological abnormalities found in chronic schizophrenia. These are well summarized by Siever & Davies [13]. Patients suffering from SzPD are also known to display deficits in cognitive-perceptual and interpersonal disturbances, together with disorganized speech and behaviour that have been viewed as a premorbid or prodromal stage of schizophrenia [30, 31]. The genetic, cognitive and neurobiological basis of overlap between schizoid personality disorders, schizotypal personality disorders and schizophrenia are well described by Ettinger et al. [32] and most recently by Schultze-Lutter et al. [33]

Due to the phenomenological similarity of symptoms in paranoid personality disorder (PPD) such as suspiciousness and paranoid delusion with schizophrenia, PPD appears to have much in common with schizophrenia. However, the evidence for this association is not strong. Akhtar [34] synthesized the descriptive and psychodynamic features of PPD in an insightful article and suggests that an important feature of the PPD is a discrepancy between the outer persona and the inner world of such individuals [34]. The author cites the work of Lowenthal [35] and Bergman [36, 37] who studied the outcome of paranoid personality during middle and old age. They suggest that the fighting stance of paranoid personalities keeps them intact; failure is never their own. Their life presents a diverting struggle against dangerous external forces and there is little time for despair and depression. This is confirmed to some extent in a relatively sparse literature on the longitudinal course of PPD. Johnson et al. [38] showed that PPD traits decline by 46% from adolescence to early adulthood [38].

5.3 Cluster A Personality Disorders and Clinically High-Risk States for Psychosis

Much research and clinical work over the last two decades have focused on the pre-psychotic or “prodromal” stages of illness. This pre-psychotic stage is characterized by increasing changes in thinking, feeling and behaving from a person’s premorbid mental state and level of functioning up to the appearance of psychotic features [12]. A number of criteria have been described to diagnose these states. Two well-defined criteria for diagnosing the high-risk states before the onset of psychosis have been developed and tested. These include the Ultra-High Risk (UHR) and the Basic Symptom (BS) criteria [39].

The criteria developed for these high-risk states have a number of symptoms that are found in patients with cluster A personality disorders. In particular symptoms of schizotypal personality disorder such as unusual thought contents or magical thinking are included in these instruments [33, 40, 41]. Racioppi et al. [42] showed that schizotypy predicted psychotic-like symptoms, depression, low self-esteem and was related to schizophrenia-spectrum [42]. The overlap between cluster A personality disorders and clinical high-risk states is illustrated in Table 5.1.

Table 5.1 Common features between cluster A personality disorders and high-risk states prior to onset of schizophrenia

High-risk states prior to onset of schizophrenia	Clinical features shared with cluster A Personality Disorders
Clinical high-risk for psychosis (CHRP)	• Ideas of reference[a] • Odd beliefs or magical thinking[a] • Perceptual disturbances[a] • Odd thinking and speech[a] • Paranoid ideation[b] • Hallucination • Delusions[a] • Formal thought disorder • Thought interference/ preservation/ pressure/blockage • Disturbance of speech / abstract thinking[a] • Decreased ability to discriminate between ideas and perceptions[a] • Derealization • Inability to divide attention • Taking substances regularly • Decrease in mental functioning
At risk for mental state (ARMS)	• Unusual thoughts[a] • Delusional mood and feeling perplexed • Bizarre ideas (being controlled by someone else)[a] • Ideas of reference (ideas that things happening around you have a significant meaning)[a] • Suspiciousness, persecutory ideas[b] • Ideas of guilt, being punished for doing something wrong • Jealous ideas[a] • Disorganized speech[a] • Aggressive/dangerous behaviour[a] • Suicidal and self-injurious behaviour
Attenuated psychotic syndrome	• Delusions/delusional ideas[b] • Hallucinations/perceptual abnormalities[a] • Disorganized speech/communication[a] • Feeling out of control of own mind • Feelings of superiority • Using odd or confusing words when you speak[a]

[a]Common in one PD in cluster A personality disorders
[b]Common in two PDs of cluster A personality disorders

Zoghbi et al. [43] examined the relationship between Attenuated Psychosis Syndrome (APS) and Schizotypal Personality Disorder, in a cohort of 218 individuals whose symptoms met APS criteria [43]. It was found that SzPD was highly prevalent (68%), and that SzPD did not influence risk for conversion to psychosis. The authors concluded that when encountering a patient whose presentation meets SzPD criteria, the clinician should assess whether APS criteria are also met and the positive symptoms are carefully monitored for possible conversion to threshold psychosis.

A recent systematic review that focused on personality disorders in patients at risk for psychosis found the prevalence of different personality disorders was quite high in these conditions, with a baseline comorbidity present in 39.4% of CHR individuals [44]. Specifically, 13.4% and 11.9% of CHR patients had comorbid Shizotypal PD and borderline PD. There were not enough studies to perform meta-analytic estimations of the prevalence rates for other personality disorders included in the cluster A personality disorders, i.e. Paranoid and Schizoid PD. Authors noticed that these prevalence rates in CHR individuals are four times greater than those in the general population. They also found that the empirical literature regarding PDs and at-risk mental states is limited, studies were heterogeneous and included a variety of different assessment measures and procedures. The lengths of follow-up periods also varied quite significantly between studies.

5.4 Interventions for Treating Cluster A Personality Disorders

This section will provide an overview of the pharmacological and non-pharmacological interventions for CAPD. Patients with these disorders often suffer from marked social and occupational impairment. They are also reluctant to engage in treatment. There is also evidence to suggest that they have unusual sensitivity to side effects. These and other factors discussed below mean that the evidence on treatment of these disorders is severely limited.

The schizotypal and schizoid personality disorders will be considered together for these interventions due to many similarities in the treatment options, while interventions for PPD will be described separately.

5.5 Pharmacological Interventions for Cluster A Personality Disorders

Pharmacological treatment in personality disorders generally tends to be symptom specific. The drug treatment usually focusses on dimensions of personality which force patients and carers to seek medical attention, and in the view of health professionals are most likely to respond to pharmacotherapy. These dimensions may be affective dysregulation (e.g. angry, anxious, depressed and elated mood), cognitive-perceptual symptoms (e.g. auditory and visual hallucinations), and impulsive aggression (e.g. self-cutting and suicidality) [45, 46]. Mostly drug treatment is adjunctive, with the goal of providing enough stabilization to make it easier or possible for the patient to engage in psychosocial interventions or overcome crisis situations. With the exception of borderline personality disorders, the evidence base for pharmacological treatments of personality disorders is fairly limited.

Various drug treatments have been used to treat different psychopathologies and symptoms associated with SzPD. These range from antipsychotics to stimulants. Antipsychotics are most commonly used drugs but antidepressants, stimulants, benzodiazepines and cognitive enhancers are also used. Medications can play either a primary or adjunctive role in treatment of patients with SPD or schizotypal traits. However, clinical trials' evidence for these personality disorders or specific schizotypal symptoms is fairly limited.

It has been suggested that attentional and cognitive difficulties are responsive to stimulants, such as those used to treat attention deficit disorder [6]. The use of stimulants in those with a vulnerability to psychosis poses the risk of exacerbation of psychotic symptoms. However, Rosell et al. [6] assert that this was not the case and on the contrary, they found that the enhanced cognitive function may limit stress-induced impairment of executive function, and therefore, lessen the propensity to more regressive forms of thought processes. These findings are based on small studies with several methodological limitations.

In a recent review, Kirchner et al. [5] identified one double-blind treatment-controlled trial; one single-blind, placebo-controlled trial; four open-label trials; one retrospective study; and four case reports on pharmacological treatment of SzPD. In total, 16 individual drug treatments were studied [5]. The most frequently studied drug was risperidone [47–50], and the most frequently studied class of drugs were the antipsychotics [47–58] followed by the antidepressants [59–61]. Six studies tested other neuroactive compounds [62–67]. In addition to differences in study designs, the included studies reporting of outcomes was not consistent. In one retrospective study, for example, Aripiprazole was used to treat all patients with schizoid, schizotypal personality and schizophrenia spectrum disorder, but no specific results were reported for SzPD [52].

Studies reported a variety of outcome measures. In most studies, the main outcome measurement was a general psychiatric symptom scale, such as the Brief Psychiatric Rating Scale [47, 52, 67], the Hopkins Symptom Checklist, and the Psychiatric Assessment Interview [58]. Three trials used interviews for specific psychotic symptoms, such as the Positive and Negative Symptom Scale (PANSS) [48, 49, 66]. Some studies focused on patients with comorbidities of OCD or Borderline Personality Disorders (BPD) and consequently measured outcomes with the Yale-Brown Obsessive Compulsive Scale (YBOCS) [51, 53, 56, 59] or the Self-Injurious Behaviour scale [54]. One study used a specific tool, the SPQ, to assess the severity of STPD as an additional outcome measurement tool [48]. The common secondary outcomes were measurements for global functioning, i.e. the Global Assessment of Symptoms [47] and Clinical Global Impression [48], or for depressive symptoms, i.e. the Hamilton Rating Scale for Depression [48, 57, 59]. Six studies had cognitive measures, i.e. working memory [62, 64, 65], context processing [63], reaction time [50], response inhibition [50] or a combination of different cognitive categories [49], as a primary or secondary outcome.

Antipsychotics seemed to have a beneficial effect on the symptoms of SzPD. Risperidone has been the most commonly used drug in these studies. In a double-blind, placebo-controlled study of low-dose risperidone (0.25–2 mg), Koenigsberg et al. [48] found improvement in the PANSS score. The trial included only 25 patients and no improvement was reported in schizotypal-specific instrument SPQ [48]. In an open-label study, Rybakowski et al. [57] found an increase in social and occupational functioning and cognitive test scores after risperidone treatment [57]. McClure et al. [49] assessed the effect of Risperidone on cognitive symptoms in a double-blind placebo-controlled trial. Only 20 of 31 patients completed 10 weeks trial and there was no beneficial effect of risperidone on measurements [49]. Rabella et al. [50] reported an experimental study examining the effect of Risperidone on reaction time using different neurophysiologic measures in patients with SzPD versus normal controls. They found an improvement in reaction time after treatment with risperidone [50].

In a 26-week, open-label study with flexible dose design, a small cohort ($n = 11$) of patients with SzPD showed significant improvements in psychosis and depression ratings, as well as in overall functioning with the use of Olanzapine [47].

In other studies, antipsychotics were mainly used as augmentation strategies for conditions such as OCD and Borderline personality disorders with comorbid cluster A personality disorders. Bogetto et al. [51] reported an open-label trial of augmentation with olanzapine (5 mg/day) for patients with OCD who were receiving fluvoxamine (300 mg/day). Out of 20 patients, four patients had comorbid SzPD and this group showed improvement in obsessive-compulsive symptoms as measured by the YBOCS score [51]. Concomitant schizotypal personality disorder was the only factor significantly associated with response to Olanzapine. Similarly, in a case report, Poyurovsky [56] described the beneficial effect in two treatment-refractory OCD patients with comorbid SzPD. Relatively low doses of clozapine were well tolerated and resulted in clinically significant improvement in obsessive-compulsive symptoms as well as improvement in tardive dyskinesia [56]. Two studies investigated the use of small doses of thiothixene versus haloperidol and thiothixene vs placebo in mixed cohorts of SzPD and BPD patients [53, 54, 58]. Both studies found a better response to thiothixene compared to haloperidol and placebo. The main areas of positive response were those of cognitive disturbance, derealization, ideas of reference, anxiety and depression.

There are also few studies reporting the use of antidepressants in people with SzPD but all of these studies have a comorbid borderline personality disorder or OCD. Markovitz et al. [68] investigated the effect of Fluoxetine in 22 patients with borderline or schizotypal personality disorder in a prospective, open-label 12-week trial. There were significant reductions in self-injury and in scores on the Hopkins Symptom Checklist regardless of diagnosis [68]. In another study, Baer et al. [59] used clomipramine for inpatients with obsessive-compulsive disorder and comorbid

A personality disorders [59]. Patients with a cluster A personality disorder had significantly higher obsessive-compulsive disorder severity scores. At the end of the 12-week study, no significant difference in treatment outcome with clomipramine was found between those patients with at least one personality disorder and those with no personality disorders. The comorbid schizotypal or other personality disorders predicted poorer treatment outcomes. One case report described a patient with SzPD who developed transient psychosis with psychogenic polydipsia on fluoxetine [60]. In another case report, a patient with OCD, anorexia nervosa and SzPD showed improvement in OCD and schizotypal personality disorder starting on a combination of paroxetine with an antipsychotic [61].

The following pharmacological agents have been evaluated for improving cognitive functions in patients with SzPD: dopamine and norepinephrine agonist d-amphetamine, D1 receptor agonist dihydrexidine, cholinesterase inhibitor physostigmine and an α_{2A} receptor agonist guanfacine [62–66]. These agents were tested in double-blind randomized controlled trials and mostly found the beneficial effects of these pharmacological agents on neuropsychological performance on measures such as working and verbal memory, executive functioning and information processing. The clinical measures to record the effect on symptoms were mostly not used or these studies.

From this overview of the literature, it appears that antipsychotics are the most commonly reported pharmacological intervention for treatment of schizotypal personality disorders. The use of antipsychotics is associated with improvement in psychotic and anxiety symptoms. However, studies are small, with relatively short follow up and usually patients had other comorbid diagnoses. Rosell et al. [6] advise caution against using antipsychotics, as psychotic symptoms are not necessarily the most disturbing to patients. They suggest that antipsychotics may be helpful when SzPD patients develop brief psychotic episodes, which they are susceptible to during periods of elevated psychosocial stress [6]. The quality of evidence for antidepressant use in SPD and SzPD is poor and is limited to open-label studies in patients with comorbid OCD and borderline PD. The published literature suggests that antidepressants may either be ineffective or perhaps associated with a risk of exacerbation in psychotic symptoms. The drug treatment to improve cognitive functions in SzPD is still in an experimental stage limited to a few studies with very small sample sizes and generally studies appear to have high risk of bias.

The paranoid personality disorder appears to have received the least attention in research relative to other personality disorders in cluster A personality disorders. The literature is limited to few case studies or case series or uncontrolled studies.

Birkeland [69] reported a case series describing the treatment of 15 patients in Denmark with paranoid personality disorder. Clinical Global Impression was rated at first admission, at the last psychiatric visit, and after a 6-week observation period with or without antipsychotic treatment. In total, seven patients had been administered any antipsychotic medication. The most commonly prescribed antipsychotic was flupenthixol. Only four patients who received antipsychotic medication could be reviewed at the 6-week follow-up. All four of these patients demonstrated improvement as measured by the Clinical Global Impression Improvement scale.

Additionally, of the 10 patients who were not lost to follow-up, antidepressant medications had been administered to a total of seven patients. Only three patients demonstrated benefit as measured by a decrease in depression symptoms. Authors concluded that antipsychotics appeared to be safe and possibly had an effect in the short term [69].

5.5.1 Non-pharmacological Interventions for Cluster A Personality Disorders

There is hardly any evidence base for psychological interventions to treat these personality disorders. Most studies are limited to case reports and individual therapists' experience of treating schizotypal and schizoid patients based on psychodynamic observations.

In a useful review, Rosell et al. [6] identified several challenges in providing psychotherapy for patients with SzPD. These include (a) limited capacity or desire to form a therapeutic alliance, (b) during the treatment patient may experience a blurring of the boundaries between themselves and the therapist, (c) Patients may not be able to tolerate regular or extended periods of separation and (d) they may have difficulty in experiencing continuity between sessions—as if the work of each session was not cumulative, but rather, was just another 'new' session (e) peculiarities of thought and semantic processing in SzPD sometimes make it very difficult for patients to be understood and/or communicate complex emotional and psychological states and concepts that are typically required in psychotherapy. It was noted by the authors that patients with SzPD exhibit a striking capacity for disavowal of certain realities, which further complicates the process of psychotherapy as the anxiety associated with certain external consequences plays less of a motivating role for psychological change. These challenges and symptoms of SzPD such as vivid perceptual/dissociative disturbance and magical beliefs require a delicate psychotherapeutic approach in patients with SzPD. The therapists face a dual challenge; being able to tolerate the anxieties of working with these phenomena and also help the patient tolerate these complicated and troubling experiences.

Stone [70] provides a highly useful account of clinical experience in treating schizotypal patients It is noted that empirical studies are lacking in part due to fact that the term schizotypal personality disorder was not found in literature before 1980 and patients are rarely seen in hospital settings. The author illustrates the challenges and approach that can be useful in one-to-one psychotherapy with schizotypal and schizoid patients [70] by using case vignettes from his own clinical practice and advice from psychodynamic literature, such as classical studies by Vanggaard [71], Nacht [72], Mosher & Gunderson [73] and Kahut [74]. The author stresses that psychotherapy of patients with schizotypal personality requires some adaptations. A summary of important points in working with schizotypal and schizoid patients is provided below.

Treating schizoid or schizotypal personality disorders is regarded as a long-term commitment, likely to last many years. The principal aim of psychotherapy in this group of patients is to help the patient to have feelings, emotions, and experiences they were incapable of having before therapy. This is fostered through the patient–therapist relationship. Therapists may need to adopt a more "active" approach and greater attention to countertransference. He points out that these patients stir up much stronger countertransference feelings in therapists.

A particular 'atmosphere' or 'climate', which is described by Guntrip [75] as 'nonverbal healing ambience' is required in therapy. This atmosphere is analogous to the 'atmosphere' of the living room where mother is *there,* watching the play of her young child, who scarcely notices her presence, and yet who derives from that unobtrusive presence, the comfort, and sense of encouragement from the mother. Whereas a correct interpretation can lead to insight, the creation of the proper relationship creates a good feeling, more akin to touching, which is central to the success of therapy in schizoid and schizotypal PD.

Ego-boundary problems are often intense in this population. Therapeutic measures that may prove helpful in dealing with ego boundary problems include appropriate limit-setting, strict punctuality about time and duration of sessions, and a decisive and firm-bordered expressions in the therapy. The interpretation of the *content* in therapy sessions should be avoided or carefully done. It is argued that the content interpretations at best might be superfluous, given the schizotype's familiarity with his incestuous, homosexual, murderous and other primitive fantasies; at worst, it might intensify the patient's already great burden of shame concerning these fantasies. Aggressive interpretation of such material may precipitate psychotic breakdown.

The Ullevål Personality Project in Norway evaluated 114 patients in an RCT [76]. In this trial, Combined Psychotherapy (CP) which consisted of a combination of psychodynamic and cognitive behavioural group therapies was compared with outpatient individual psychotherapy (OIP). Patients with schizotypal PD and antisocial PD were excluded. Paranoid and schizoid personality disorders comprised 15% and 1% of all personality disorder diagnoses, respectively. The data for specific personality types was not reported but there was no interaction between specific PD criteria and outcome in the two treatment arms. The main finding was that the more intensive, multimodal combined psychotherapy (CP) was not more beneficial in terms of efficacy than outpatient individual psychotherapy (OIP). In fact, psychosocial functioning from 18 months to 3 years exhibited a significantly more favourable course in the outpatient treatment group [76]. Interestingly 6 years follow-up of the cohort [77] showed that patients in the outpatient group had a marked decline in psychosocial functioning during the period between the 3- and 6-year follow-ups; while psychosocial functioning continued to improve in the combined psychotherapy group during the same period.

One clinical trial [78] compared integrated therapy with the standard treatment to prevent transition to psychosis for first-contact patients with schizotypal disorder (as defined in ICD-10). The integrated treatment comprised interventions such as social skills training, psychoeducation and assertive community treatment. The integrated treatment inhibited or postponed transition to psychotic disorder better than standard treatment, However, a substantial proportion of patients also received antipsychotics in the intervention group, so the effects of treatment could not be attributed to psychosocial interventions alone.

An uncontrolled prospective study [79] of day hospital therapeutic community treatment found 'very modest' improvement for schizotypal disorder patients. A case report by McKay & Neziroglu [80] described the treatment of a person with obsessive-compulsive disorder and schizotypal personality using social skills training. At 6-month follow-up, the patient had considerable improvement in obsessive-compulsive symptoms as well as symptoms of anxiety and depression as measured by relevant and validated scales.

Psychotherapeutic approaches can be particularly challenging for paranoid PD in view of suspiciousness and hostility being cardinal features of the disorder. Freud theorized that paranoia is an externalizing defence against unconscious homosexual wishes [81] though there has been little theoretical or empirical support for the idea. The psychoanalytic approaches have been used in treatment of PPD. However, in cases accepted for psychoanalysis, the symptoms are less severe and the diagnosis of BPD is often comorbid with BPD [82].

In theory, cognitive approaches may suit for the treatment of PPD, since these may help to ameliorate the cognitive distortions associated with paranoid thinking. Systematic data are lacking regarding the effectiveness but case reports show potential effectiveness [83, 84]. One such case report found cognitive analytic therapy to be an effective intervention [83]. Data from intensive psychotherapeutic day treatment programmes showed that paranoid personality disorder is a significant predictor of treatment failure and drop out, irrespective of the PPD being a diagnosis on its own or comorbid with borderline PD [79, 85].

5.6 Challenges and Opportunities for Research and Treatment of Cluster A Personality Disorder

It is clear that cluster A personality disorders have a long history which is deeply rooted in the concept of schizophrenia and psychosis in general. The disorders have been part of the classification systems in one way or another for at least five decades. However, the research on psychopathology, the relationship between psychosis and treatment has lagged behind in comparison to other personality disorders such as borderline PD. It is noteworthy, for example, that evidence-based recommendations are still lacking for the diagnosis and treatment of personality disorders included in this cluster.

NICE (National Institute for Health and Care Excellence, UK) which produces guidelines on all important aspects of health care only has produced guidelines for borderline and antisocial PD. None of the research recommendations formulated by NICE for treatment and prevention of schizophrenia (https://www.nice.org.uk/guidance/cg178/evidence/full-guideline-490503565) includes the research on these or other personality disorders that can be precursor to psychosis onset. In a review of guidelines from European countries, Simonsen et al. [86] concluded that clinical guidelines for PD treatment almost exclusively focussed on BPD [86]. Only the

World Federation of Societies of Biological Psychiatry (WFSBP) provided guidelines on treatment of schizotypal PD and recommended that there is low-quality evidence for use of antipsychotics in reducing symptom severity in this PD [87] but these guidelines need updating. This is a major challenge. As we have discussed above, the quality of evidence for such guidelines may not be high but producing guidelines and identifying the gaps in knowledge will help research and clinicians in this field.

A major challenge is to bridge the gap between the research on these disorders and recently emerging concepts such as CHR or At Risk Mental State (ARMS). We believe the emergence of these concepts such as 'clinically high risk states for psychosis' have contributed to relative lack of understanding and have eclipsed the research effort in cluster A personality disorders. These concepts undoubtedly led to a large body of research and helped in developing the services for early intervention in psychosis. However, the At Risk Mental State (ARMS) or CHR has a large degree of overlap with cluster A personality disorders. Cluster A personality disorders are included in the existing classification systems while these newer concepts are still not part of the official classification systems, with the exception of the recent inclusion of Attenuated Psychosis Syndrome (APS) in DSM-5. Unsurprisingly perhaps the domains such as CHR or APS had little clinical influence beyond the highly specialized research and early intervention services.

It should be possible to investigate the cluster A personality disorders and At Risk Mental State at the same time in view of significant overlap between these conditions. A major challenge is to include the assessment for these disorders in early intervention in psychosis programmes that are already using a wide range of assessment tools for assessing psychosis risk. This can help to better understand the prodrome to the onset of psychosis. Few studies have attempted this approach. Zhang et al. [88], for example used a screening questionnaire to examine the prevalence of SzPD in people with clinical high risk (CHR) state and found that identifying SzPD may be useful in the early detection of psychosis in those at high risk of psychosis. In the context of an intensive early intervention programme (OPUS), Nordentoft et al. [78] investigated the effect of integrated treatment on the transition to psychosis in those diagnosed with schizotypal disorder. They reported the beneficial effects of the intensive treatment consisting of assertive outreach, family involvement, and social skills training in preventing the transition to psychosis at 2 years follow up, although the effect was not sustained at 3.5 years follow-up period [89].

Improving the tools for screening and diagnosing these personality disorders can help to detect those who may be at higher risk of developing psychosis, especially if these can be integrated with existing prodromal screen tools. Salokangas et al. [90] found that the schizotypal personality questionnaire and items describing ideas of reference and lack of close interpersonal relationships correlated significantly with the transition to psychosis.

An important challenge is to conduct adequately powered intervention trials in this population who are very difficult to engage. The evidence for efficacy of interventions for management of cluster A personality disorders is limited. The evidence for treatment of SzPD is relatively better compared to other disorders in the cluster but even here it is limited to one double-blind and one single-blind placebo-controlled trial. These trials are not adequately powered. An important outcome to measure would be the transition to psychosis.

5.7 Conclusions

Personality disorders included in cluster A represent a major group of personality disorders that are relatively common. These personality disorders are responsible for high burden of disease, disability and can potentially be precursors to schizophrenia. In particular, schizotypal and schizoid PDs in this cluster share a long history with the concept of schizophrenia and have a number of neurobiological and phenomenological similarities with schizophrenia and related psychosis. In clinical samples defined by schizotypal disorder (as defined by ICD-10), schizoid or Schizotypal personality disorder, up to 48% developed psychosis [40]. Paranoid personality disorders share a number of phenomenological similarities with schizophrenia but the evidence of transition to psychosis is not as strong.

The personality disorders in this cluster have a well-established tradition, rich literature on aetiology, pathophysiology and phenomenology and are recognized in two major classification systems, i.e. ICD-10 and DSM-V. However, over the last two decades much of the research attention has been given to ARMS and related concepts as precursors to schizophrenia. Despite extensive research into psychosis prevention based on understanding the aetiology, pathophysiology and phenomenology of at-risk mental states and clinically high-risk states for psychosis, there has been limited success in preventing transition to psychosis. In a recent systematic review and meta-analysis [91] included a total of 128 original controlled studies that investigated the evidence for risk and protective factors for developing psychosis in Clinical High Risk for Psychosis (CHR-P). The authors retrieved and evaluated 26 factors and concluded that 'our findings suggest that despite the large number of putative risk factors investigated in the literature, only attenuated positive psychotics symptoms, global functioning, and negative psychotics symptoms show suggestive evidence or greater for association with transition to psychosis. It is noteworthy that all three factors mentioned here feature in cluster A personality disorders and an approach integrating these personality disorders may yield better dividends.

The early detection and treatment of these personality disorders may potentially help to prevent the transition to psychosis and complement the present research efforts in CHR states. The research in early detection and treatment of psychosis is now well established and has identified many potential pathways for preventing or delaying the onset of psychosis. We believe integrating the assessment and treatment of cluster A personality disorders with early intervention in psychosis will inform both treatments of schizophrenia and personality disorders.

References

1. American Psychiatric Association, American Psychiatric Association, & DSM-5 Task Force. (2013). *Diagnostic and statistical manual of mental disorders: DSM-5*. http://dsm.psychiatryonline.org/book.aspx?bookid=556
2. World Health Organization. International classification of diseases 10th edition (ICD 10) research diagnostic criteria. World Health Organization; 1993. http://www.who.int/classifications/icd/en/
3. World Health Organization. International classification of diseases for mortality and morbidity statistics. World Health Organization; 2018. https://icd.who.int/browse11/l-m/en
4. Bach B, First MB. Application of the ICD-11 classification of personality disorders. BMC Psychiatry. 2018;18(1):351. https://doi.org/10.1186/s12888-018-1908-3.
5. Kirchner SK, Roeh A, Nolden J, Hasan A. Diagnosis and treatment of schizotypal personality disorder: evidence from a systematic review. NPJ Schizophr. 2018;4(1):20. https://doi.org/10.1038/s41537-018-0062-8.
6. Rosell DR, Futterman SE, McMaster A, Siever LJ. Schizotypal personality disorder: a current review. Curr Psychiatry Rep. 2014;16(7):452. https://doi.org/10.1007/s11920-014-0452-1.
7. Barrantes-Vidal N, Grant P, Kwapil TR. The role of schizotypy in the study of the etiology of schizophrenia spectrum disorders. Schizophr Bull. 2015;41(Suppl 2):S408–16. https://doi.org/10.1093/schbul/sbu191.
8. Bateman AW, Gunderson J, Mulder R. Treatment of personality disorder. Lancet. 2015;385(9969):735–43. https://doi.org/10.1016/S0140-6736(14)61394-5.
9. Carroll A. Are you looking at me? Understanding and managing paranoid personality disorder. Adv Psychiatr Treat. 2009;15(1):40–8. https://doi.org/10.1192/apt.bp.107.005421.
10. Torgersen S, Kringlen E, Cramer V. The prevalence of personality disorders in a community sample. Arch Gen Psychiatry. 2001;58(6):590–6. https://doi.org/10.1001/archpsyc.58.6.590.
11. Grant BF, Hasin DS, Stinson FS, Dawson DA, Chou SP, Ruan WJ, Pickering RP. Prevalence, correlates, and disability of personality disorders in the United States: results from the national epidemiologic survey on alcohol and related conditions. J Clin Psychiatry. 2004;65(7):948–58. https://doi.org/10.4088/jcp.v65n0711.
12. Yung AR, McGorry PD. The initial prodrome in psychosis: descriptive and qualitative aspects. Aust N Z J Psychiatry. 1996;30(5):587–99. https://doi.org/10.3109/00048679609062654.
13. Siever LJ, Davis KL. The pathophysiology of schizophrenia disorders: perspectives from the spectrum. Am J Psychiatry. 2004;161(3):398–413. https://doi.org/10.1176/appi.ajp.161.3.398.
14. Tyrer P, Gunderson J, Lyons M, Tohen M. Extent of comorbidity between mental state and personality disorders. J Personal Disord. 1997;11(3):242–59. https://doi.org/10.1521/pedi.1997.11.3.242.
15. Fonseca Pedrero E, Debbané M. Schizotypal traits and psychotic-like experiences during adolescence: an update. Psicothema. 2017;29(1):5–17. https://doi.org/10.7334/psicothema2016.209.
16. Bleuler E. *Dementia Praecox or the Group of Schizophrenias* (J. Zinkin translation). International Universities Press; 1911.
17. Flückiger R, Michel C, Grant P, Ruhrmann S, Vogeley K, Hubl D, Schimmelmann BG, Klosterkötter J, Schmidt SJ, Schultze-Lutter F. The interrelationship between schizotypy, clinical high risk for psychosis and related symptoms: cognitive disturbances matter. Schizophr Res. 2019;210:188–96. https://doi.org/10.1016/j.schres.2018.12.039.
18. Flückiger R, Ruhrmann S, Debbané M, Michel C, Hubl D, Schimmelmann BG, Klosterkötter J, Schultze-Lutter F. Psychosis-predictive value of self-reported schizotypy in a clinical high-risk sample. J Abnorm Psychol. 2016;125(7):923–32. https://doi.org/10.1037/abn0000192.
19. Lenzenweger MF. Schizotypy, schizotypic psychopathology, and schizophrenia: hearing echoes, leveraging prior advances, and probing New angles. Schizophr Bull. 2018a;44(suppl_2):S564–9. https://doi.org/10.1093/schbul/sby083.
20. Lenzenweger MF. Schizotypy, schizotypic psychopathology and schizophrenia. World Psychiatry. 2018b;17(1):25–6. https://doi.org/10.1002/wps.20479.

21. Michel C, Flückiger R, Kindler J, Hubl D, Kaess M, Schultze-Lutter F. The trait-state distinction between schizotypy and clinical high risk: results from a one-year follow-up. World Psychiatry. 2019;18(1):108–9. https://doi.org/10.1002/wps.20595.
22. Cohen AS, Chan RCK, Debbané M. Crossing boundaries in schizotypy research: an introduction to the special supplement. Schizophr Bull. 2018;44(suppl_2):S457–9. https://doi.org/10.1093/schbul/sby089.
23. Laguerre A, Leboyer M, Schürhoff F. The schizotypal personality disorder: historical origins and current status. L'Encephale. 2008;34(1):17–22. https://doi.org/10.1016/j.encep.2007.07.007.
24. Lenzenweger MF. Schizotypy and schizophrenia: the view from experimental psychopathology. Guilford Press; 2010.
25. Lenzenweger MF. Thinking clearly about schizotypy: hewing to the schizophrenia liability core, considering interesting tangents, and avoiding conceptual quicksand. Schizophr Bull. 2015;41(Suppl 2):S483–91. https://doi.org/10.1093/schbul/sbu184.
26. Kendler KS, McGuire M, Gruenberg AM, O'Hare A, Spellman M, Walsh D. The Roscommon family study. III. Schizophrenia-related personality disorders in relatives. Arch Gen Psychiatry. 1993;50(10):781–8. https://doi.org/10.1001/archpsyc.1993.01820220033004.
27. Kety SS, Wender PH, Jacobsen B, Ingraham LJ, Jansson L, Faber B, Kinney DK. Mental illness in the biological and adoptive relatives of schizophrenic adoptees. Replication of the Copenhagen study in the rest of Denmark. Arch Gen Psychiatry. 1994;51(6):442–55. https://doi.org/10.1001/archpsyc.1994.03950060006001.
28. Kendler KS, Gruenberg AM, Tsuang MT. Psychiatric illness in first-degree relatives of schizophrenic and surgical control patients. A family study using DSM-III criteria. Arch Gen Psychiatry. 1985;42(8):770–9. https://doi.org/10.1001/archpsyc.1985.01790310032004.
29. Tsuang MT, Stone WS, Tarbox SI, Faraone SV. An integration of schizophrenia with schizotypy: identification of schizotaxia and implications for research on treatment and prevention. Schizophr Res. 2002;54(1–2):169–75. https://doi.org/10.1016/s0920-9964(01)00364-4.
30. Bedwell JS, Donnelly RS. Schizotypal personality disorder or prodromal symptoms of schizophrenia? Schizophr Res. 2005;80(2–3):263–9. https://doi.org/10.1016/j.schres.2005.07.023.
31. Raine A. Schizotypal personality: neurodevelopmental and psychosocial trajectories. Annu Rev Clin Psychol. 2006;2:291–326. https://doi.org/10.1146/annurev.clinpsy.2.022305.095318.
32. Ettinger U, Meyhöfer I, Steffens M, Wagner M, Koutsouleris N. Genetics, cognition, and neurobiology of schizotypal personality: a review of the overlap with schizophrenia. Front Psych. 2014;5:18. https://doi.org/10.3389/fpsyt.2014.00018.
33. Schultze-Lutter F, Nenadic I, Grant P. Psychosis and schizophrenia-Spectrum personality disorders require early detection on different symptom dimensions. Front Psych. 2019;10:476. https://doi.org/10.3389/fpsyt.2019.00476.
34. Akhtar S. Paranoid personality disorder: a synthesis of developmental, dynamic, and descriptive features. Am J Psychother. 1990;44(1):5–25. https://doi.org/10.1176/appi.psychotherapy.1990.44.1.5.
35. Lowenthal MF. The relationship between social factors and mental health in the aged. In: Simon A, Epstein LJ, editors. Aging in modern society. Am Psychiatr Assoc. Washington, DC; 1968. pp. 187–97.
36. Bergman K. The neuroses of old age. In: Kay DW, Walk A, editors. Recent developments in psychogeriatrics. Br J Psychiatry; 1971. p. 39–50.
37. Bergman K. Neurosis and personality disorder in old age. In: Issacs AD, Post F, editors. Studies in geriatric psychiatry. John Wiley; 1978. p. 41–76.
38. Johnson JG, Cohen P, Kasen S, Skodol AE, Hamagami F, Brook JS. Age-related change in personality disorder trait levels between early adolescence and adulthood: a community-based longitudinal investigation. Acta Psychiatr Scand. 2000;102(4):265–75. https://doi.org/10.1034/j.1600-0447.2000.102004265.x.
39. Fusar-Poli P, McGorry PD, Kane JM. Improving outcomes of first-episode psychosis: an overview. World Psychiatry. 2017;16(3):251–65. https://doi.org/10.1002/wps.20446.
40. Debbané M, Eliez S, Badoud D, Conus P, Flückiger R, Schultze-Lutter F. Developing psychosis and its risk states through the lens of schizotypy. Schizophr Bull. 2015;41(Suppl 2):S396–407. https://doi.org/10.1093/schbul/sbu176.

41. Schultze-Lutter F, Schimmelmann BG, Ruhrmann S, Michel C. 'A rose is a rose is a rose', but at-risk criteria differ. Psychopathology. 2013;46(2):75–87. https://doi.org/10.1159/000339208.
42. Racioppi A, Sheinbaum T, Gross GM, Ballespí S, Kwapil TR, Barrantes-Vidal N. Prediction of prodromal symptoms and schizophrenia-spectrum personality disorder traits by positive and negative schizotypy: a 3-year prospective study. PLoS One. 2018;13(11):e0207150. https://doi.org/10.1371/journal.pone.0207150.
43. Zoghbi AW, Bernanke JA, Gleichman J, Masucci MD, Corcoran CM, Califano A, Segovia J, Colibazzi T, First MB, Brucato G, Girgis RR. Schizotypal personality disorder in individuals with the attenuated psychosis syndrome: frequent co-occurrence without an increased risk for conversion to threshold psychosis. J Psychiatr Res. 2019;114:88–92. https://doi.org/10.1016/j.jpsychires.2019.04.018.
44. Boldrini T, Tanzilli A, Pontillo M, Chirumbolo A, Vicari S, Lingiardi V. Comorbid personality disorders in individuals with an at-risk mental state for psychosis: a meta-analytic review. Front Psych. 2019;10:429. https://doi.org/10.3389/fpsyt.2019.00429.
45. Binks CA, Fenton M, McCarthy L, Lee T, Adams CE, Duggan C. Pharmacological interventions for people with borderline personality disorder. Cochrane Database Syst Rev. 2006;1:CD005653. https://doi.org/10.1002/14651858.CD005653.
46. Soloff PH. Algorithms for pharmacological treatment of personality dimensions: symptom-specific treatments for cognitive-perceptual, affective, and impulsive-behavioral dysregulation. Bull Menn Clin. 1998;62(2):195–214.
47. Keshavan M, Shad M, Soloff P, Schooler N. Efficacy and tolerability of olanzapine in the treatment of schizotypal personality disorder. Schizophr Res. 2004;71(1):97–101. https://doi.org/10.1016/j.schres.2003.12.008.
48. Koenigsberg HW, Reynolds D, Goodman M, New AS, Mitropoulou V, Trestman RL, Silverman J, Siever LJ. Risperidone in the treatment of schizotypal personality disorder. J Clin Psychiatry. 2003;64(6):628–34. https://doi.org/10.4088/jcp.v64n0602.
49. McClure MM, Koenigsberg HW, Reynolds D, Goodman M, New A, Trestman R, Silverman J, Harvey PD, Siever LJ. The effects of risperidone on the cognitive performance of individuals with schizotypal personality disorder. J Clin Psychopharmacol. 2009;29(4):396–8. https://doi.org/10.1097/JCP.0b013e3181accfd9.
50. Rabella M, Grasa E, Corripio I, Romero S, Mañanas MÀ, Antonijoan RM, Münte TF, Pérez V, Riba J. Neurophysiological evidence of impaired self-monitoring in schizotypal personality disorder and its reversal by dopaminergic antagonism. NeuroImage Clin. 2016;11:770–9. https://doi.org/10.1016/j.nicl.2016.05.019.
51. Bogetto F, Bellino S, Vaschetto P, Ziero S. Olanzapine augmentation of fluvoxamine-refractory obsessive-compulsive disorder (OCD): a 12-week open trial. Psychiatry Res. 2000;96(2):91–8. https://doi.org/10.1016/s0165-1781(00)00203-1.
52. Di Lorenzo R, Amoretti A, Forghieri M, Fiorini F, Genedani S, Rigatelli M. Aripiprazole: effectiveness and safety under naturalistic conditions. Exp Clin Psychopharmacol. 2007;15(6):569–75. https://doi.org/10.1037/1064-1297.15.6.569.
53. Goldberg SC, Schulz SC, Resnick RJ, Hamer RM, Schulz PM. Differential prediction of response to thiothixene and placebo in borderline and schizotypal personality disorders. Psychopharmacol Bull. 1987;23(3):342–6.
54. Goldberg SC, Schulz SC, Schulz PM, Resnick RJ, Hamer RM, Friedel RO. Borderline and schizotypal personality disorders treated with low-dose thiothixene vs placebo. Arch Gen Psychiatry. 1986;43(7):680–6. https://doi.org/10.1001/archpsyc.1986.01800070070009.
55. Hymowitz P, Frances A, Jacobsberg LB, Sickles M, Hoyt R. Neuroleptic treatment of schizotypal personality disorders. Compr Psychiatry. 1986;27(4):267–71. https://doi.org/10.1016/0010-440x(86)90001-5.
56. Poyurovsky M. Clozapine in treatment-refractory obsessive-compulsive disorder with comorbid schizotypal personality disorder. Isr J Psychiatry Relat Sci. 2008;45(3):219–20.
57. Rybakowski JK, Dròzdz W, Borkowska A. Low dose risperidone in the treatment of schizophrenia-like symptoms in high-risk subjects. J Clin Psychopharmacol. 2003;23(6):674–5. https://doi.org/10.1097/01.jcp.0000095352.32154.e1.

58. Serban G, Siegel S. Response of borderline and schizotypal patients to small doses of thiothixene and haloperidol. Am J Psychiatry. 1984;141(11):1455–8. https://doi.org/10.1176/ajp.141.11.1455.
59. Baer L, Jenike MA, Black DW, Treece C, Rosenfeld R, Greist J. Effect of axis II diagnoses on treatment outcome with clomipramine in 55 patients with obsessive-compulsive disorder. Arch Gen Psychiatry. 1992;49(11):862–6. https://doi.org/10.1001/archpsyc.1992.01820110026003.
60. Gutkovich Z, Rosenthal RN, Bogdonoff L. Transient psychosis with psychogenic polydipsia in schizotypal patient taking fluoxetine. Psychosomatics. 1998;39(3):295–6. https://doi.org/10.1016/S0033-3182(98)71349-0.
61. Heiden A, de Zwaan M, Frey R, Presslich O, Kasper S. Paroxetine in a patient with obsessive-compulsive disorder, anorexia nervosa and schizotypal personality disorder. J Psychiatry Neurosci. 1998;23(3):179–80.
62. Kirrane RM, Mitropoulou V, Nunn M, Silverman J, Siever LJ. Physostigmine and cognition in schizotypal personality disorder. Schizophr Res. 2001;48(1):1–5. https://doi.org/10.1016/s0920-9964(00)00059-1.
63. McClure MM, Barch DM, Romero MJ, Minzenberg MJ, Triebwasser J, Harvey PD, Siever LJ. The effects of guanfacine on context processing abnormalities in schizotypal personality disorder. Biol Psychiatry. 2007;61(10):1157–60. https://doi.org/10.1016/j.biopsych.2006.06.034.
64. McClure MM, Harvey PD, Goodman M, Triebwasser J, New A, Koenigsberg HW, Sprung LJ, Flory JD, Siever LJ. Pergolide treatment of cognitive deficits associated with schizotypal personality disorder: continued evidence of the importance of the dopamine system in the schizophrenia spectrum. Neuropsychopharmacology. 2010;35(6):1356–62. https://doi.org/10.1038/npp.2010.5.
65. Rosell DR, Zaluda LC, McClure MM, Perez-Rodriguez MM, Strike KS, Barch DM, Harvey PD, Girgis RR, Hazlett EA, Mailman RB, Abi-Dargham A, Lieberman JA, Siever LJ. Effects of the D1 dopamine receptor agonist dihydrexidine (DAR-0100A) on working memory in schizotypal personality disorder. Neuropsychopharmacology. 2015;40(2):446–53. https://doi.org/10.1038/npp.2014.192.
66. Siegel BV, Trestman RL, O'Flaithbheartaigh S, Mitropoulou V, Amin F, Kirrane R, Silverman J, Schmeidler J, Keefe RS, Siever LJ. D-amphetamine challenge effects on Wisconsin Card Sort Test. Performance in schizotypal personality disorder. Schizophr Res. 1996;20(1–2):29–32. https://doi.org/10.1016/0920-9964(95)00002-x.
67. Zwier KJ, Rao U. Buspirone use in an adolescent with social phobia and mixed personality disorder (cluster A type). J Am Acad Child Adolesc Psychiatry. 1994;33(7):1007–11. https://doi.org/10.1097/00004583-199409000-00011.
68. Markovitz PJ, Calabrese JR, Schulz SC, Meltzer HY. Fluoxetine in the treatment of borderline and schizotypal personality disorders. Am J Psychiatry. 1991;148(8):1064–7. https://doi.org/10.1176/ajp.148.8.1064.
69. Birkeland SF. Psychopharmacological treatment and course in paranoid personality disorder: a case series. Int Clin Psychopharmacol. 2013;28(5):283–5. https://doi.org/10.1097/YIC.0b013e328363f676.
70. Stone M. Schizotypal personality: psychotherapeutic aspects. Schizophr Bull. 1985;11(4):576–89. https://doi.org/10.1093/schbul/11.4.576.
71. Vanggaard T. Borderlands of sanity. Munksgaard; 1979.
72. Nacht S. The non-verbal relationship in psycho-analytic treatment. Int J Psychoanal. 1963;44:328–33.
73. Mosher LR, Gunderson JG. Group, family, milieu, and community-support-systems treatment for schizophrenia. In: Bellak L, editor. Disorders of the schizophrenic syndrome. Basic Books; 1979. p. 399–452.
74. Kahut H. Analysis of the self. International Universities Press; 1971.
75. Guntrip H. The schizoid compromise and psychotherapeutic stalemate. Br J Med Psychol. 1962;35:273–87. https://doi.org/10.1111/j.2044-8341.1962.tb00525.x.
76. Arnevik E, Wilberg T, Urnes Ø, Johansen M, Monsen JT, Karterud S. Psychotherapy for personality disorders: 18 months' follow-up of the ullevål personality project. J Personal Disord. 2010;24(2):188–203. https://doi.org/10.1521/pedi.2010.24.2.188.

77. Antonsen BT, Kvarstein EH, Urnes Ø, Hummelen B, Karterud S, Wilberg T. Favourable outcome of long-term combined psychotherapy for patients with borderline personality disorder: six-year follow-up of a randomized study. Psychother Res. 2017;27(1):51–63. https://doi.org/10.1080/10503307.2015.1072283.
78. Nordentoft M, Thorup A, Petersen L, Ohlenschlaeger J, Melau M, Christensen TØ, Krarup G, Jørgensen P, Jeppesen P. Transition rates from schizotypal disorder to psychotic disorder for first-contact patients included in the OPUS trial. A randomized clinical trial of integrated treatment and standard treatment. Schizophr Res. 2006;83(1):29–40. https://doi.org/10.1016/j.schres.2006.01.002.
79. Karterud S, Vaglum S, Friis S, Irion T, Johns S, Vaglum P. Day hospital therapeutic community treatment for patients with personality disorders. An empirical evaluation of the containment function. J Nerv Ment Dis. 1992;180(4):238–43. https://doi.org/10.1097/00005053-199204000-00005.
80. Mckay D, Neziroglu F. Social skills training in a case of obsessive-compulsive disorder with schizotypal personality disorder. J Behav Ther Exp Psychiatry. 1996;27(2):189–94. https://doi.org/10.1016/0005-7916(96)00010-9.
81. Freud S. *Pscyho-analytic notes upon an autobiographical account of a case of paranoia (dementia paranoides)* (standard edition). Hogarth Press; 1911.
82. Lee R. Mistrustful and misunderstood: a review of paranoid personality disorder. Curr Behav Neurosci Rep. 2017;4(2):151–65. https://doi.org/10.1007/s40473-017-0116-7.
83. Kellett S, Hardy G. Treatment of paranoid personality disorder with cognitive analytic therapy: a mixed methods single case experimental design. Clin Psychol Psychother. 2014;21(5):452–64. https://doi.org/10.1002/cpp.1845.
84. Nicolo G, Centerno E, Nobile S, Porcari F. Paranoid personality disorder: a single case intervention. Ric Psicoter. 2003;5:89–107.
85. Kvarstein EH, Karterud S. Large variations of global functioning over five years in treated patients with personality traits and disorders. J Personal Disord. 2012;26(2):141–61. https://doi.org/10.1521/pedi.2012.26.2.141.
86. Simonsen S, Bateman A, Bohus M, Dalewijk HJ, Doering S, Kaera A, Moran P, Renneberg B, Ribaudi JS, Taubner S, Wilberg T, Mehlum L. European guidelines for personality disorders: past, present and future. Borderline Personal Disord Emot Dysregul. 2019;6(1):9. https://doi.org/10.1186/s40479-019-0106-3.
87. Herpertz SC, Zanarini M, Schulz CS, Siever L, Lieb K, Möller H-J. WFSBP Task Force on Personality Disorders. World Federation of Societies of Biological Psychiatry (WFSBP) guidelines for biological treatment of personality disorders. World J Biol Psychiatry. 2007;8(4):212–44. https://doi.org/10.1080/15622970701685224.
88. Zhang T, Li H, Tang Y, Li H, Zheng L, Guo Q, Zhao S, Zhuo K, Qian Z, Wang L, Dai Y, Chow A, Li C, Jiang K, Wang J, Xiao Z. Screening schizotypal personality disorder for detection of clinical high risk of psychosis in Chinese mental health services. Psychiatry Res. 2015;228(3):664–70. https://doi.org/10.1016/j.psychres.2015.04.049.
89. Albert N, Glenthøj LB, Melau M, Jensen H, Hjorthøj C, Nordentoft M. Course of illness in a sample of patients diagnosed with a schizotypal disorder and treated in a specialized early intervention setting. Findings from the 3.5year follow-up of the OPUS II study. Schizophr Res. 2017;182:24–30. https://doi.org/10.1016/j.schres.2016.10.013.
90. Salokangas RKR, Dingemans P, Heinimaa M, Svirskis T, Luutonen S, Hietala J, Ruhrmann S, Juckel G, Graf von Reventlow H, Linszen D, Birchwood M, Patterson P, Schultze-Lutter F, Klosterkötter J, EPOS group. Prediction of psychosis in clinical high-risk patients by the schizotypal personality questionnaire. Results of the EPOS project. Eur Psychiatry. 2013;28(8):469–75. https://doi.org/10.1016/j.eurpsy.2013.01.001.
91. Oliver D, Reilly TJ, Baccaredda Boy O, Petros N, Davies C, Borgwardt S, McGuire P, Fusar-Poli P. What causes the onset of psychosis in individuals at clinical high risk? A meta-analysis of risk and protective factors. Schizophr Bull. 2020;46(1):110–20. https://doi.org/10.1093/schbul/sbz039.

6 Risk Factors of Early Onset of Borderline Personality Disorder: A Conceptual Model

Silvio Bellino, Marco Bosia, Cristiana Montemagni, Paola Rocca, and Paola Bozzatello

6.1 Borderline Personality Disorder: A Complex Diagnosis

Borderline Personality Disorder (BPD) is a distressing and multifaceted mental disorder characterized by a pervasive pattern of instability in interpersonal relationships, self-image, and affects, and marked impulsivity that is expressed in a variety of contexts [1]. In the traditional psychoanalytic setting, individuals who were particularly resistant to treatment were defined "borderline" as they were thought to occupy a "border" between "psychotic" and "neurotic" disorders. The criteria for BPD were originally defined by Spitzer and colleagues in 1979 in an effort to determine what clinical features characterized patients who were referred to as "borderline." These authors described a psychopathological pattern reflecting instability of affect, identity disturbance, and deficiency of impulse control. The most common pattern of clinical manifestations includes chronic instability since early adolescence, with episodes of abrupt mood fluctuations and severe impulsive dyscontrol, leading to a serious impairment of interpersonal relationships and vocational functioning. BPD produces a significant dysfunction of self-regulation in the social context and both affective instability and catastrophic reactions to the loss of emotionally invested social ties position BPD in the area of attachment disorders. Proceeding from Bowlby's theory [2], other Authors suggested that intolerance of aloneness and inability to invoke a "soothing introject" in BPD patients were consequences of early attachment failures [3, 4]. In particular, an insecure disorganized attachment

S. Bellino (✉) · M. Bosia · C. Montemagni ·P. Rocca · P. Bozzatello
Department of Neuroscience "Rita Levi Montalcini", University of Turin, Turin, Italy
e-mail: silvio.bellino@unito.it; marco.bosia@unito.it; cristiana.montemagni@unito.it; paola.rocca@unito.it; paola.bozzatello@unito.it

P. Rocca, S. Bellino (eds.), *Psychosis and Personality Disorders*,
https://doi.org/10.1007/978-3-031-09058-5_6

with parental figures may generate in these patients a particular vulnerability to turmoil and challenges at a later time [5, 6].

The heterogeneity of psychopathology and clinical course of BPD has impeded efforts to produce hypotheses on aetiopathogenesis of the disorder, as well as to identify biomarkers and endophenotypes [7]. Despite problems with heterogeneity, data from family and twin studies, longitudinal investigations, and biological research suggest that BPD is a meaningful clinical construct that deserves to be furtherly refined [8].

In young subjects, epidemiological data indicate a point prevalence of around 0.9%, but clinical studies in this age group are still limited. Cumulative prevalence rates of BPD in adolescents are respectively 1.4% and 3.2% at 16 years and at 22 years. In psychiatric contexts, prevalence increases to 11% in outpatients and even to 50% in patients admitted to hospital [9]. According to the literature data, long-term impairment is originated by early onset of BPD symptomatology and some core features of the disorder persist for up to 20 years. Despite the fact that this personality disorder emerges and develops during adolescence, diagnosis is often delayed since clinicians are hesitant to make this serious diagnosis in teenagers because of such issues as difficulties in distinguishing personality disorder from physiological developmental crises, and the risk of stigma and prejudice. Nevertheless, it is very important to make an early diagnosis in order to deliver early interventions and significantly improve clinical outcomes and quality of life. Delaying the diagnosis and treatment of BPD has noticeable negative implications for patients, as evidences are accumulating that many of the psychopathological disturbances associated with BPD emerge early in the course of the disorder and delay in intervention is likely to cause worse functional impairment. These evidences support the recommendations provided by recent treatment guidelines for BPD [10, 11]. Although early identification of BPD in young patients is needed and can improve the prognosis of the disorder, it could be deceiving to talk about "adolescent BPD": this personality disorder maintains the same structure across lifetime, with a peak incidence in adolescence and early adulthood that subsequently declines partly due to maturational or socialization processes. To improve the process of early diagnosis and intervention, a fundamental issue is the recognition of risk factors and precursors of BPD. In recent years, several antecedents of the disorder have been identified and described in clinical studies. In particular, some precocious environmental factors, child and adolescent temperamental traits, early psychopathological characteristics, and neurobiological correlates appear to play a crucial role in the development of BPD and they will be the object of the following paragraphs.

6.2 Environmental Factors

A broad range of environmental factors that have been related to increasing risk for BPD were identified and proposed in literature, including socioeconomic status, family psychopathology, parent–child relationship, and maltreatments or other traumatic events in early life. In recent years, a growing number of investigations have been also focused on the effects of bullying and rejection by peer groups in the onset of BPD.

There is general accordance among clinicians and investigators that early circumstances and environmental factors play a fundamental and primary role in the development of BPD. Among family-related environmental factors, low family socioeconomic status, confirmed by assessment of low income, low educational level, and low occupational status and indirectly by the access to public assistance, prepares for early BPD onset. Some studies on large samples followed for a period ranged between 10 and 20 years [12–14] suggested that low socioeconomic status of the family of origin appears to be an independent prospective risk factor for the development of severe personality disorders (such as BPD and schizotypal personality disorder) and observed that family access to public assistance predicted the onset of BPD symptomatology. Low socioeconomic status seems to be linked with the tendency of parents to show a large amount of expressed emotion. Thus, economical environmental conditions together with maladaptive behaviours in parents are two prospective risk factors for early BPD [14–16].

Another risk factor we should take into account when considering early onset of BPD is maternal psychopathology. The most robust data concern the association between maternal BPD and offspring early BPD [17–19]. Maternal borderline symptoms are linked to a particular kind of parenting, known as psychological control, in which mothers manipulate offspring's emotions and their expressions. Maternal psychological control was related to the affective imbalance of adolescents, which leads to an increased risk of developing BPD themselves [17, 18, 20]. Rejection and overprotection are two key features of mothers' dysfunctional behaviour and alternation between these two attitudes makes it impossible for children to understand and foresee how their mothers would behave. The association between other maternal psychopathological conditions, such as maternal externalizing disorders (conduct disturbances, oppositional defiant disorder, attention-deficit/hyperactivity disorder, impulsive-aggressive behaviours, self-injuries, and substance use disorder) and internalizing disorders (depression and anxiety, dissociation, and suicidality) with early BPD onset is still understudied. In a longitudinal study carried out on a high-risk community sample of 700 youth followed from mid-adolescence to young adulthood [21], maternal internalizing disorders were not related to offspring BPD development, whereas maternal externalizing disorders showed the strongest impact out of all risk factors on adolescent BPD symptoms, but there was no one-to-one relationship between maternal and adolescent BPD symptoms, confirming the conceptual model that no risk factor on its own can cause BPD. Nevertheless, other Authors reported that also maternal internalizing disorder during pregnancy could be a risk factor for BPD development in offspring, in particular, prenatal anxiety and depression were significantly associated with BPD offspring at 11–12 years old [22, 23].

As concerns the relationships between parents and children, some kinds of dysfunctional parent–child relationships were identified as a potential predictor of early BPD: discord between mother and child, roles confusion and disoriented behaviours in parents, inadequate parent–child boundaries, psychological control by parents, and low relationships quality in individuals with a particular genotype for the oxytocin receptor gene [21, 24–27]. In line with the environment–genes interactions' theory, patients with a specific genotype seem to be more sensitive to environmental stressors and prone to BPD development [28]. For example, a polymorphism of the oxytocin receptor gene, involved in socioemotional functioning, interacted with quality of family relationships to foster borderline personality disorder (BPD) symptomatology in a sample of 20-year-old subjects [28]. Adolescents with an AA/AG genotype appear more sensitive to familial relationship quality. Those with the AA/AG genotype who grow up in families characterized by low discord develop few or no BPD symptoms. On the other hand, when raised in families with high levels of familial discord, young people with this genotype express clinically significant borderline pathology. Adolescents with a GG genotype seem to be less sensitive to familial relationship quality and develop average levels of BPD symptoms regardless of reported level of interpersonal discord [28]. Gene–environment interaction is particularly important in BPD expression also as regards precocious traumatic experiences. Traumatic events, especially early trauma, play a central role in the development of BPD as they impair the skill of mentalizing or symbolizing emotions. Verbal abuse, emotional abuse, physical abuse, sexual abuse, emotional and physical neglect, and chronic exposure to peer victimization were identified as potential risk factors for young BPD [14, 18, 26, 29–40]. Although it remains to be further studied and better understood how genetic factors may interact with the environmental factors in promoting precocious BPD symptoms, some authors suggested that subjects with particular gene polymorphisms of oxytocin receptor and FK506 binding protein have a greater risk to develop BPD in presence of early maltreatment experiences [41].

6.3 Temperament and Personality Traits

In order to recognize predictors of BPD at the early phases of life, investigation of intrapsychic factors is needed, including temperamental characteristics and personality traits in adolescence, which could increase the risk of early onset of this disorder. Studies that were conducted on this focus suggested that several personality traits in children or adolescents, including affective instability, negative affectivity, negative emotionality, inappropriate anger, poor emotional control, impulsivity, and aggression, could prepare for borderline pathology [38, 39, 42, 43]. Few studies evaluated the relationship of childhood personality traits to BPD in adulthood [31, 44, 45], while a good number of investigations evaluated the relationship between temperament or personality features associated with early BPD symptoms [38–40, 43, 46–52].

Authors that adopted Cloninger's model of temperament and character to investigate the association between temperamental patterns in childhood or adolescence and onset of BPD, reported that high harm avoidance, high novelty seeking, and low reward dependence represent a pattern of biological vulnerability for developing BPD [46, 50]. Other temperamental traits that were found associated to precocious BPD were aggressiveness, in particular relational aggression [38, 40, 43, 48], affective instability, and negative affectivity [14, 42, 47, 53–56]. Low level of self-control and impulsivity can be considered predictors of borderline pathology in young age [57, 58]. Vaillancourt et al. [43] reported some gender differences in the associations between temperamental traits and onset of BPD: relational aggression was the predominant predictor in boys, while physical aggression was the strongest predictor in girls.

Moreover, some temperamental features seem to interact with familial environment in producing BPD in early age. In fact, some evidences supported that low emotional control, negative affectivity, and low affiliation in adolescence may produce an early onset of BPD by association with parental maltreatment, harsh discipline, and familial adversities [15, 16, 30, 59]. One study investigated the interaction of a temperamental risk factor and a neurobiological risk factor in predicting the emergence of BPD during early adolescence, examining several temperamental factors and volumetric measures of hippocampal asymmetry. Results showed that subjects were more likely to develop BPD symptoms in presence of high affiliation, low effortful control, and rightward hippocampal asymmetry [52].

6.4 Early Psychopathological Features

BPD onset can be anticipated by several psychopathological characteristics emerging during childhood and adolescence. Internalizing disorders consist of psychopathological syndromes that cause inner suffering to the individual, such as depression, anxiety, dissociation, and suicidality, whereas externalizing disorders are characterized by dysfunctional behaviours manifested outside and performed against others, including oppositional defiant disorder, conduct disturbances, attention-deficit/hyperactivity disorder (ADHD), impulsive-aggressive behaviours, and substance use disorder. Both internalizing and externalizing disorders represent a predisposing condition to the early development of BPD when associated to biological vulnerabilities and environmental factors [31, 42, 60].

Several studies found that depression, among internalizing disorders, is associated with early onset of borderline psychopathology [19, 21, 42, 59, 61–63]. A recent study performed by Sharp et al. [59] on a large sample of adolescents, showed that anxiety and depression at young age were associated to borderline features via experiential avoidance (EA), a specific construct conceived as "unwillingness to remain in contact with uncomfortable private events, such as thoughts, emotions, sensations, memories, and urges." The Authors hypothesized that EA could be considered as an underlying psychological process of all three mental disorders and observed that EA predicted levels of borderline symptoms. Association between other internalizing disorders, such as dissociation [63], self-injuries [64], and suicidality [19], and early BPD symptoms are less studied and requires further assessment to draw any conclusion.

A reasonable amount of studies have also identified the influence of externalizing disorders over paving the way to early onset of BPD. ADHD in both childhood [65, 66] and adolescence [62, 67] increases the risk of developing BPD early adulthood. Oppositional defiant disorder and conduct disorder were found positively associated to early BPD display [19, 66–68] and could share with ADHD the same pathogenic process that fosters this personality disorder.

In addition, substance use disorder can be considered a predictive factor of early onset of BPD [19, 61, 62].

Some authors suggested that psychopathology emerges in pre-adolescence in the form of anxiety and depressive symptoms in females, while it is more commonly represented by ADHD and conduct problems in males. These disorders may form a substrate on which personality pathology takes shape during adolescence [60, 69]. These antecedent psychopathologies could represent a predisposing condition that interacts with stressful life events and, if untreated, contribute to the onset of personality pathology during adolescence [60]. An additional hypothesis to explain the overlap of internalizing and externalizing disorders is that BPD pathology expresses itself in early stages of the disorder mainly with externalizing behaviours, although features of internalizing disorders are also present. During adulthood, behavioural manifestations of externalizing disorders are usually replaced by a stronger expression of internalizing pathology [57, 58, 70].

6.5 Brain Imaging Findings in Early-Onset BPD

Studies of neuroimaging in BPD patients in adolescence could allow to understand how brain's morphology and function appear at the beginning of the disorder, before course of illness, extended use of medications, and accumulated traumas modify cerebral structures and activity [71]. Unfortunately, to date, these investigations in young patients are still scarce and concern only structural studies. Trials performed on adult BPD found abnormalities in the frontolimbic structures, including volume reductions in the amygdala [72, 73], hippocampus [72, 73], orbitofrontal cortex (OFC) [74], frontal lobes [75], and cingulate cortex [74, 76]. These structural findings are matched with functional alterations, in particular, the increased reactivity of areas accountable for emotional processing, including insula, hippocampus, and amygdala, and the decreased recruitment of regulatory control regions, involving anterior cingulate cortex (ACC), medial frontal cortex (MFC), OFC and dorsolateral prefrontal cortex (DLPFC) [77, 78].

In adolescent BPD patients, consistently with findings obtained in adult subjects, it was observed a significant reduction in volume of OFC [79–81] and ACC [82, 83] compared with healthy controls. Findings concerning the hippocampus and amygdala are more controversial. In fact, some studies reported no differences between BPD young patients and healthy controls in the volume of these areas [79–81], whereas other investigations found an atypical rightward hippocampal asymmetry associated with specific temperamental traits in BPD adolescents, such as high affiliation and low effortful control [30], and a volume shrinking of both right amygdala and hippocampus in youths with BPD in comparison with healthy controls [71]. Also in white matter, some specific alterations were observed: white matter tracts connecting parts of the limbic system to the OFC [84] and bilateral fornices [85] showed a diminished fractional anisotropy in BPD adolescents compared with controls. Although functional studies of brain imaging have not been carried out yet in young subjects with BPD, these findings regarding the white matter are similar to those obtained from functional studies conducted in BPD adults [86], that display a disruption in frontolimbic system connectivity accountable for dysfunctional emotion processing.

6.6 Early Treatments

Interventions in adolescence require caution as it is a critical period during which characteristics of BPD are flexible and fluid and differential diagnosis is often uncertain, but as soon as symptoms of BPD are definitely distinguished from physiological turmoil of adolescence, adequate early treatments are necessary to obtain better results to counteract the chronicity and functional impairment of the disorder with its negative consequences, such as polypharmacy and frequent hospitalizations. In adult BPD patients, a growing number of evidences on efficacy of medications and psychotherapies have been collected, but no medication has obtained an official indication to treat this disorder, yet [57, 58]. Nevertheless, systematic reviews and guidelines for the treatment of adult BPD were published to orient the psychiatrists in clinical practice [10, 11, 87–90]. Among pharmacotherapies, mood stabilizers (valproate, topiramate and lamotrigine), antipsychotics of second generation (olanzapine and quetiapine) and third generation (aripiprazole), and new agents, such as omega-3 fatty acids, are the compounds that acquired more robust evidences of efficacy, but medications are targeted on specific symptom domains (affective instability, impulsive behavioural dyscontrol, cognitive-perceptual symptoms) and no pharmacotherapy can actually be indicated to deal with the global psychopathology of this personality disorder [57, 58]. In fact, several core symptom domains, such as fears of abandonment, chronic feelings of emptiness, and identity disturbances are refractory to pharmacotherapy and should be investigated as the target of specific psychotherapies or combined therapies.

Several psychotherapeutic approaches were specifically developed or adapted for BPD patients. Most investigated models of psychotherapy in adults were dialectical behaviour therapy (DBT) [91] among cognitive-behavioural therapies, and mentalization-based therapy [92] among psychodynamic treatments. Initial evidences were recently obtained concerning the adaptation of interpersonal psychotherapy to BPD (IPT-BPD) [93–96].

While in adult BPD patients some evidences of efficacy were obtained for specific treatments, studies on therapies for young patients are not sufficient and we have rather embryonic data. Basic principles of early intervention in young subjects with BPD should be represented by an appropriate diagnostic approach, which consists of an accurate diagnosis made with criteria that allow a stratification of subsyndromal and full-syndromal BPD, and by effective treatment strategies, based on the fundamental components of general psychiatric care and individual psychotherapy, involvement of families and caretakers, supervision of staff members, and a social perspective which considers educational and work purposes [9]. Treatment of adolescents with BPD needs a high level of commitment from both patients and their families. As it happens for adults, polypharmacy is often used in adolescents to target specific symptom domains, although there are no clinical evidences to endorse the use of medications, which should be restricted to the treatment of acute crises and comorbidities. According to data available in adults, second-generation antipsychotics could be administered during acute crises and anxiolytics in a short period [97]. The only randomized controlled trial on pharmacological treatment for adolescents with BPD is a 12-week double-blind randomized controlled trial (RCT) that compared long-chain omega-3 polyunsaturated fatty acids (PUFAs) (1.2 g/day) with placebo in a group of BPD adolescents with ultra-high risk for psychosis [98]. Trial reported that omega-3 fatty acids are useful to improve functioning and to reduce psychiatric symptoms.

Some models of psychotherapy validated in adults were adapted for adolescents, but data of efficacy are still limited. Available studies have tested the Cognitive Analytic Therapy (CAT), the Dutch Emotion Regulation Training (ERT) treatment programme, the Mentalization-Based Treatment for Adolescents (MBT-A), the Dialectical Behaviour Therapy for Adolescents (DBT-A), and the Transference-Focused Psychotherapy (TFP).

CAT is a time-limited psychotherapy developed by Ryle [99] from the integration of psychoanalytical-oriented object relations theory and cognitive approach. It focuses on understanding of maladaptive patient's behaviour in order to let him acknowledge dysfunctional patterns and find different strategies to deal with stressful situations. It is the first evidence-based treatment tested in the context of the Helping Young People Early (HYPE) programme in Melbourne, a specific service conceived to offer prevention and early intervention [100, 101]. The routine treatment consists of a maximum of 24 sessions and 4 follow-up meetings which monitor the progression. CAT displays a practical and collaborative style, with a particular focus on identifying, understanding, and revising the individual's problematic self-management and interpersonal relationship patterns and the thoughts, feelings, and behavioural responses that result from these patterns. A typical feature in CAT is the joint (patient therapist) creation of a shared understanding of the patient's issues and their developmental origins, using narrative and diagrammatic "reformulations" written in plain language. In the RCT performed by Chanen [81], outpatients aged with BPD between 15 and 18 years were randomly assigned to either CAT or manualized Good Clinical Care (GCC). Both treatments were equally effective at the 2-year follow-up assessment, although CAT was associated with more rapid improvement of internalizing and externalizing symptoms. The Authors performed a subsequent quasi-experimental study [100, 101] to compare these two treatments to historical treatment as usual (TAU) and found that GCC and CAT were more effective than TAU at reducing psychopathology and parasuicidal behaviours and at improving global functioning.

ERT is a 17-session, manual-based, group-based skills training and individual and family psychoeducation programme [102]. It was developed from Systems Training for Emotional Predictability and Problem Solving (STEPPS) for adult BPD [103]. It combines cognitive behavioural elements and skills training with a systemic component. In a RCT [104] assessing young people with BPD, aged 14–19 years, assigned to ERT + TAU or TAU alone, both groups showed improvement on primary measures of mood regulation and borderline symptomatology after 6 months, with no differential effects between groups. So, initial data were not in favour of ERT as augmentation strategy in young BPD patients.

Mentalization-Based Treatment for Adolescents (MBT-A) is a psychodynamic psychotherapy derived from Bateman and Fonagy's MBT for adults [105] on the basis of attachment theory and is delivered as a one-year-long programme including weekly individual MBT sessions and monthly mentalization-based family therapy. Its final goal is to improve the ability to understand mental states and behaviours in oneself and others. In the RCT carried out by Rossouw & Fonagy [106], a sample of 12–17-year-old adolescents (85% females) with borderline symptomatology (73% of them met full BPD criteria) and self-reported depression were randomly assigned to either MBT-A or "treatment as usual" (TAU). Outcomes displayed that MBT-A was more effective than TAU in reducing BPD symptoms, self-mutilation, and depression. The positive effect of MBT-A on self-mutilating behaviour was mediated by an improvement in mentalization and attachment abilities. A second RCT [107] tested the efficacy of MBT in groups (MBT-G) in adolescents aged between 14 and 17 years, randomized to a one-year MBT-G or TAU with at least 12 monthly individual sessions. MBT-G consists of three introductory, psychoeducational sessions, 37 weekly group sessions, five individual case formulation sessions, and six group sessions for caregivers, and represents a less costly approach than individual psychotherapy. The results showed no superiority of either therapy method, with a considerable amount of drop out in MBT-G group. It can be suggested that individual MBT is more promising than group MBT to treat adolescents with BPD, although a direct comparison should be performed.

Dialectical Behaviour Therapy for Adolescents (DBT-A) was developed from Linehan's DBT for adults [91]. It combines elements of cognitive-behavioural therapy with awareness and relaxation techniques from the Zen Buddhism. It is delivered over 19 weeks and comprises weekly individual psychotherapy sessions, weekly multifamily skills training, family therapy sessions, and telephone coaching. Skills training groups are one of the most well-known features of DBT, conveying practical skills for the improvement of stress tolerance, emotion regulation, interpersonal difficulties, and awareness to individuals with BPD. In addition to adult DBT, the integration of families is a central component of DBT-A. Mehlum and colleagues conducted a RCT [108] and a 1-year follow-up study [109] in a sample of adolescents (mean age = 15.6 years) who were assigned to either DBT-A or Enhanced Usual Care (EUC) group (weekly psychodynamically oriented therapy or CBT). The 1-year follow-up assessment demonstrated a stronger long-term reduction in self-harms and a more rapid recovery in suicidal ideation, depression, and borderline symptoms in the DBT-A group.

Transference-focused psychotherapy is a psychoanalytic psychotherapy approach that was developed by Kernberg and his group in accordance with object relations theory [110]. It combines classic psychoanalytic techniques with a more structured and presence-focused approach that fits the needs of patients with BPD. The transference-focused psychotherapy has been manualized and adapted for the treatment of adolescent BPD (adolescent identity treatment): the primary modifications of TFP for adolescent treatment involve changes in frequency and duration of some of the specific techniques, such as increased clarification, extra-transferential relationships before directly addressing the transference, inclusion of family during the assessment phase, and treatment contract setting phases of treatment. To our knowledge, data on the efficacy of TFP for adolescents are not available, yet.

The majority of treatment strategies discussed above, except for ERT and MBT-G, produced an effect on BPD symptoms. However, the manualized interventions, such as CAT, MBT-A, DBT-A, and also GCC, were found superior to usual care programmes, TAU or EUC, in improving some specific BPD symptoms (e.g. self-harms) and global functioning, and in terms of time needed to observe these improvements.

6.7 A Conceptual Model of Risk Factors for Early-Onset BPD

On the basis of the findings presented in the previous paragraphs, adolescence has to be considered a vulnerable phase for the development of BPD. It is important to detect the main risk factors linked to onset of BPD in this period of life in order to monitor high-risk population since premorbid manifestations. Although strong evidences support the advantages in terms of outcome of early identification of BPD, fear of stigma for young people still contributes to postpone the diagnosis in clinical practice [9, 111]. Results of studies on the impact of early onset of BPD on later functioning of patients are generally in accordance to retain that BPD in adolescence predicts a severe impairment of interpersonal and occupational functioning, as well as younger age at first treatment, affective instability, antisocial behaviours, substance abuse, and dysfunctional relationships with parents. Furthermore, poor functional outcome persists up to 20 years into the future in individuals who presented BPD onset in adolescence [22, 23, 112–115].

As we have described, development of BPD symptoms in adolescence and early adulthood is associated with several clinical, temperamental, and environmental factors. Because of the high number of potential risk factors for early BPD identified in the literature, it is difficult to apply these knowledge in clinical practice, particularly in obtaining a better prevention of BPD pathology.

In order to suggest which can be the more significant risk factors and how they are associated in the clusters of environmental precocious situations, child and adolescent temperament and personality traits, early psychopathological features, and correlates of neuroimaging we propose a hypothetic model of a high-risk condition for the onset of BPD (Fig. 6.1). This model, aimed to detect early clinical conditions and to implement preventive interventions, is a combination of more relevant and common factors identified in literature and is supported by the idea that their interactive effects are stronger and more important than the separate effects of each single factor.

(1) Among family-related environmental factors, low socioeconomic status of family, economic adversities, and maladaptive behaviours in parents are three robust precursors for early BPD, together with maternal BPD psychopathology. Moreover, some dysfunctional parent–child relationships were found as potential risk factors for early onset of BPD: discord between mother and child, significant role confusion and disoriented behaviours in parents, inadequate parent–child boundaries, psychological control by parents and low relationships quality in individuals with a particular genotype for the oxytocin receptor gene. (2) Among trauma-related environmental factors, verbal, emotional, physical, and sexual abuse, emotional and physical neglect, and long-lasting exposure to peer victimization were identified as potential predictive factors for young BPD. (3) As regards child and adolescent temperamental related factors, the main predictors of early BPD were aggressiveness (in particular relational aggression), impulsivity, affective instability, negative affectivity, and low emotional control by interaction with maltreatments. (4) Psychopathological conditions during childhood and adolescence that potentially promote early onset of BPD were both internalizing (depression, anxiety, dissociation, self-harming) and externalizing disorders (substance use disorder, ADHD, opposite defiant disorder, conduct disorder). (5) Results from neuroimaging studies suggested that a reduction in

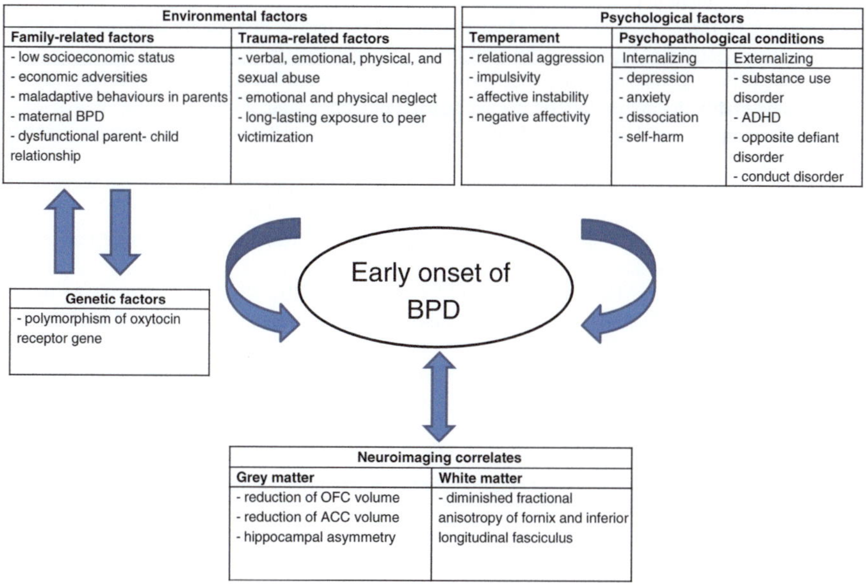

Fig. 6.1 Risk factors of early-onset borderline personality disorder

volume of OFC, ACC, and hippocampal asymmetry were observed in early BPD compared with controls. Also, some specific alterations in white matter were found: the inferior longitudinal fasciculus and the fornix showed a diminished fractional anisotropy in BPD adolescents compared with controls.

Our proposal of conceptual model is based on the evidence of literature and is characterized by the interaction of the following factors: high-risk subjects have experienced abuse/neglect in childhood and/or they have a mother with severe psychopathology; they present temperamental traits of impulsive aggression and negative affectivity interacting with dysfunctional familial environment; they display in childhood/adolescence precocious disorders such as depression, ADHD, and substances use; and they show structural abnormalities of frontolimbic areas involved in impulsive and emotional regulation [57, 58].

Of course, these indicators of a high-risk condition for early BPD onset, and the effects of their coexistence and interaction in the proposed model must be carefully investigated and supported by further and more conclusive empirical findings.

References

1. American Psychiatric Association. Diagnostic and statistical manual of mental disorders. 5th ed. Washington, DC; 2013.
2. Bowlby J. Attachment. In: Attachment and loss, vol. 1. New York: Basic Books; 1969.
3. Gunderson JG. The borderline patient's intolerance of aloneness: insecure attachments and therapist availability. Am J Psychiatry. 1996;153(6):752–8.
4. Lyons-Ruth K, Bronfman E, Atwood G. A relational diathesis model of hostile-helpless states of mind: expressions in mother-infant interaction. In: Attachment disorganization. NY: Solomon J, George C. Guilford press; 1999.
5. Fonagy P, Target M, Gergely G. Attachment and borderline personality disorder. A theory and some evidence. Psychiatr Clin North Am. 2000;23(1):103–22. vii-viii
6. Oldham JM, Skodol AE, Bender DS, editors. The American Psychiatric Publishing textbook of personality disorders. American Psychiatric Publishing, Inc; 2005.
7. Gottesman II, Gould TD. The endophenotype concept in psychiatry: etymology and strategic intentions. Am J Psychiatry. 2003;160(4):636–45.
8. Paris J. Neurobiological dimensional models of personality: a review of the models of Cloninger, Depue, and Siever. J Personal Disord. 2005;19(2):156–70.
9. Kaess M, Brunner R, Chanen AM. Borderline personality disorder in adolescence. Pediatrics. 2014;134(4):782–93.
10. National Institute for Health and Clinical Excellence (NICE). *Borderline personality disorder: treatment and management. Clinical Guideline* 78. London, UK: National Collaborating Centre for Mental Health; 2009.
11. National Health and Medical Research Council. Clinical practice guideline for the management of borderline personality disorder. Melbourne: National Health and Medical Research Council; 2012.
12. Cohen P, Chen H, Gordon K, Johnson J, Brook J, Kasen S. Socioeconomic background and the developmental course of schizotypal and borderline personality disorder symptoms. Dev Psychopathol. 2008;20(2):633–50.
13. Crawford T, Cohen P, Chen H, Anglin D, Ehrensaft M. Early maternal separation and the trajectory of borderline personality disorder symptoms. Dev Psychopathol. 2009;21(3):1013–30.
14. Stepp SD, Keenan K, Hipwell AE, Krueger RF. The impact of childhood temperament on the development of borderline personality disorder symptoms over the course of adolescence. Borderline Personal Disord Emot Dysregul. 2014a;1(1):18.

15. Stepp SD, Lazarus SA, Byrd AL. A systematic review of risk factors prospectively associated with borderline personality disorder: taking stock and moving forward. Personal Disord Theory Res Treat. 2016a;4:316–23.
16. Stepp SD, Scott LN, Jones NP, Whalen DJ, Hipwell AE. Negative emotional reactivity as a marker of vulnerability in the development of borderline personality disorder symptoms. Dev Psychopathol. 2016b;28(1):213–24.
17. Reinelt E, Stopsack M, Aldinger M, Ulrich I, Grabe HJ, Barnow S. Longitudinal transmission pathways of borderline personality disorder symptoms: from mother to child? Psychopathology. 2014;47(1):10–6.
18. Barnow S, Aldinger M, Arens EA, Ulrich I, Spitzer C, Grabe HJ, Stopsack M. Maternal transmission of borderline personality disorder symptoms in the community-based Greifswald family study. J Personal Disord. 2013;27(6):806–19.
19. Stepp SD, Olino TM, Klein DN, Seeley JR, Lewinsohn PM. Unique influences of adolescent antecedents on adult borderline personality disorder features. Personal Disord. 2013;4(3):223–9.
20. Mahan RM, Kors SB, Simmons ML, Macfie J. Maternal psychological control, maternal borderline personality disorder, and adolescent borderline features. Personal Disord. 2018;9(4):297–304.
21. Conway CC, Hammen C, Brennan PA. Adolescent precursors of adult borderline personality pathology in a high-risk community sample. J Personal Disord. 2015;29(3):316–33.
22. Winsper C, Wolke D, Lereya T. Prospective associations between prenatal adversities and borderline personality disorder at 11-12 years. Psychol Med. 2015a;45(5):1025–37.
23. Winsper C, Marwaha S, Lereya ST, Thompson A, Eyden J, Singh SP. Clinical and psychosocial outcomes of borderline personality disorder in childhood and adolescence: a systematic review. Psychol Med. 2015b;45(11):2237–51.
24. Bradley B, DeFife JA, Guarnaccia C, Phifer J, Fani N, Ressler KJ, Westen D. Emotion dysregulation and negative affect: association with psychiatric symptoms. J Clin Psychiatry. 2011;72(5):685–91.
25. Greenfield B, Henry M, Lis E, Slatkoff J, Guilé JM, Dougherty G, Zhang X, Raz A, Eugene Arnold L, Daniel L, Mishara BL, Koenekoop RK, de Castro F. Correlates, stability and predictors of borderline personality disorder among previously suicidal youth. Eur Child Adolesc Psychiatry. 2015;24(4):397–406.
26. Lyons-Ruth K, Brumariu LE, Bureau JF, Hennighausen K, Holmes B. Role confusion and disorientation in young adult-parent interaction among individuals with borderline symptomatology. J Personal Disord. 2015;29(5):641–62.
27. Vanwoerden S, Kalpakci A, Sharp C. The relations between inadequate parent-child boundaries and borderline personality disorder in adolescence. Psychiatry Res. 2017;257: 462–71.
28. Hammen C, Bower JE, Cole SW. Oxytocin receptor gene variation and differential susceptibility to family environment in predicting youth borderline symptoms. J Personal Disord. 2015;29(2):177–92.
29. Lyons-Ruth K, Bureau JF, Holmes B, Easterbrooks A, Brooks NH. Borderline symptoms and suicidality/self-injury in late adolescence: prospectively observed relationship correlates in infancy and childhood. Psychiatry Res. 2013;206(2–3):273–81.
30. Jovev M, McKenzie T, Whittle S, Simmons JG, Allen NB, Chanen AM. Temperament and maltreatment in the emergence of borderline and antisocial personality pathology during early adolescence. J Can Acad Child Adolesc Psychiatry. 2013;22(3):220–9.
31. Bornovalova MA, Huibregtse BM, Hicks BM, Keyes M, McGue M, Iacono WJ. Tests of a direct effect of childhood abuse on adult borderline personality disorder traits: a longitudinal discordant twin design. Abnorm Psychol. 2013;122(1):180–94.
32. Valentino K, Cicchetti D, Toth SL, Rogosch FA. Mother-child play and emerging social behaviors among infants from maltreating families. Dev Psychol. 2006;42(3):474–85.
33. Wolke D, Schreier A, Zanarini MC, Winsper C. Bullied by peers in childhood and borderline personality symptoms at 11 years of age: a prospective study. J Child Psychol Psychiatry. 2012;53(8):846–55.

34. Lereya ST, Winsper C, Heron J, Lewis G, Gunnell D, Fisher HL, Wolke D. Being bullied during childhood and the prospective pathways to self-harm in late adolescence. J Am Acad Child Adolesc Psychiatry. 2013;52(6):608–18.e2.
35. Winsper C, Hall J, Strauss VY, Wolke D. Aetiological pathways to borderline personality disorder symptoms in early adolescence: childhood dysregulated behaviour, maladaptive parenting and bully victimisation. Borderline Personal Disord Emot Dysregul. 2017;4:10.
36. Haltigan JD, Vaillancourt T. Identifying trajectories of borderline personality features in adolescence: antecedent and interactive risk factors. Can J Psychiatr. 2016;61(3):166–75.
37. Antila H, Arola R, Hakko H, Riala K, Riipinen P, Kantojärvi L. Bullying involvement in relation to personality disorders: a prospective follow-up of 508 inpatient adolescents. Eur Child Adolesc Psychiatry. 2017;26(7):779–89.
38. Crick NR, Murray-Close D, Woods K. Borderline personality features in childhood: a short-term longitudinal study. Dev Psychopathol. 2005;17(4):1051–70.
39. Nelson DA, Coyne SM, Swanson SM, Hart CH, Olsen JA. Parenting, relational aggression, and borderline personality features: associations over time in a Russian longitudinal sample. Dev Psychopathol. 2014;26(3):773–87.
40. Cramer P. Childhood precursors of adult borderline personality disorder features: a longitudinal study. J Nerv Ment Dis. 2016;204(7):494–9.
41. Cicchetti D, Rogosch FA, Hecht KF, Crick NR, Hetzel S. Moderation of maltreatment effects on childhood borderline personality symptoms by gender and oxytocin receptor and FK506 binding protein 5 genes. Dev Psychopathol. 2014;26(3):831–49.
42. Belsky DW, Caspi A, Arseneault L, Bleidorn W, Fonagy P, Goodman M, Houts R, Moffitt TE. Etiological features of borderline personality related characteristics in a birth cohort of 12-year-old children. Dev Psychopathol. 2012;24(1):251–65.
43. Vaillancourt T, Brittain HL, McDougall P, Krygsman A, Boylan K, Duku E, Hymel S. Predicting borderline personality disorder symptoms in adolescents from childhood physical and relational aggression, depression, and attention-deficit/hyperactivity disorder. Dev Psychopathol. 2014;26(3):817–30.
44. Carlson EA, Egeland B, Sroufe LA. A prospective investigation of the development of borderline personality symptoms. Dev Psychopathol. 2009;21(4):1311–34.
45. Conway CC, Hipwell AE, Stepp SD. Seven-year course of borderline personality disorder features: borderline pathology is as unstable as depression during adolescence. Clin Psychol Sci. 2017;5(4):742–9.
46. Joyce PR, McKenzie JM, Luty SE, Mulder RT, Carter JD, Sullivan PF, Cloninger CR. Temperament, childhood environment and psychopathology as risk factors for avoidant and borderline personality disorders. Aust N Z J Psychiatry. 2003;37(6):756–64.
47. Tragesser SL, Solhan M, Schwartz-Mette R, Trull TJ. The role of affective instability and impulsivity in predicting future BPD features. J Personal Disord. 2007;21(6):603–14.
48. Underwood MK, Beron KJ, Rosen LH. Joint trajectories for social and physical aggression as predictors of adolescent maladjustment: internalizing symptoms, rule-breaking behaviors, and borderline and narcissistic personality features. Dev Psychopathol. 2011;23(2):659–78.
49. Gratz KL, Tull MT, Reynolds EK, Bagge CL, Latzman RD, Daughters SB, Lejuez CW. Extending extant models of the pathogenesis of borderline personality disorder to childhood borderline personality symptoms: the roles of affective dysfunction, disinhibition, and self- and emotion-regulation deficits. Dev Psychopathol. 2009;21(4):1263–91.
50. Kaess M, Resch F, Parzer P, von Ceumern-Lindenstjerna IA, Henze R, Brunner R. Temperamental patterns in female adolescents with borderline personality disorder. J Nerv Ment Dis. 2013;201(2):109–15.
51. Martín-Blanco A, Soler J, Villalta L, Feliu-Soler A, Elices M, Pérez V, Arranz MJ, Ferraz L, Alvarez E, Pascual JC. Exploring the interaction between childhood maltreatment and temperamental traits on the severity of borderline personality disorder. Compr Psychiatry. 2014;55(2):311–8.

52. Jovev M, Whittle S, Yücel M, Simmons JG, Allen NB, Chanen AM. The relationship between hippocampal asymmetry and temperament in adolescent borderline and antisocial personality pathology. Dev Psychopathol. 2014;26:275–85.
53. Lenzenweger MF, Cicchetti D. Toward a developmental psychopathology approach to borderline personality disorder. Dev Psychopathol. Fall. 2005;17(4):893–8.
54. Tragesser SL, Solhan M, Brown WC, Tomko RL, Bagge C, Trull TJ. Longitudinal associations in borderline personality disorder features: diagnostic interview for borderlines-revised (DIB-R) scores over time. J Personal Disord. 2010;24(3):377–91.
55. Hallquist MN, Hipwell AE, Stepp SD. Poor self-control and harsh punishment in childhood prospectively predict borderline personality symptoms in adolescent girls. J Abnorm Psychol. 2015;124(3):549–64.
56. Stepp SD, Lazarus SA. Identifying a borderline personality disorder prodrome: implications for community screening. Personal Ment Health. 2018;11:195–205.
57. Bozzatello P, Bellino S, Bosia M, Rocca P. Early detection and outcome of borderline personality disorder. Front Psych. 2019a;9(10):710.
58. Bozzatello P, Rocca P, De Rosa ML, Bellino S. Current and emerging medications for borderline personality disorder: is pharmacotherapy alone enough? Expert Opin Pharmacother. 2019b;21(1):47–61.
59. Sharp C, Kalpakci A, Mellick W, Venta A, Temple JR. First evidence of a prospective relation between avoidance of internal states and borderline personality disorder features in adolescents. Eur Child Adolesc Psychiatry. 2015;24(3):283–90.
60. Sharp C, Wall K. Personality pathology grows up: adolescence as a sensitive period. Curr Opin Psychol. 2018;21:111–6.
61. Ramklint M, von Knorring AL, von Knorring L, Ekselius L. Child and adolescent psychiatric disorders predicting adult personality disorder: a follow-up study. Nord J Psychiatry. 2003;57(1):23–8.
62. Thatcher DL, Cornelius JR, Clark DB. Adolescent alcohol use disorders predict adult borderline personality. Addict Behav. 2005;30(9):1709–24.
63. Krabbendam AA, Colins OF, Doreleijers TA, van der Molen E, Beekman AT, Vermeiren RR. Personality disorders in previously detained adolescent females: a prospective study. Am J Orthopsychiatry. 2015;85(1):63–71.
64. Koenig J, Brunner R, Schmidt JM, Parzer P, Resch F, Kaess M. Psychopathology and borderline personality pathology associated with lifetime self-injurious behavior in adolescent psychiatric inpatients and detainees. Z Kinder Jugendpsychiatr Psychother. 2017;45(6):441–51.
65. Miller CJ, Flory JD, Miller SR, Harty SC, Newcorn JH, Halperin JM. Childhood attention-deficit/hyperactivity disorder and the emergence of personality disorders in adolescence: a prospective follow-up study. J Clin Psychiatry. 2008;69(9):1477–84.
66. Stepp SD, Burke JD, Hipwell AE, Loeber R. Trajectories of attention deficit hyperactivity disorder and oppositional defiant disorder symptoms as precursors of borderline personality disorder symptoms in adolescent girls. J Abnorm Child Psychol. 2012;40(1):7–20.
67. Burke JD, Stepp SD. Adolescent disruptive behavior and borderline personality disorder symptoms in young adult men. J Abnorm Child Psychol. 2012;40(1):35–44.
68. Stepp SD, Whalen DJ, Scott LN, Zalewski M, Loeber R, Hipwell AE. Reciprocal effects of parenting and borderline personality disorder symptoms in adolescent girls. Dev Psychopathol. 2014b;26(2):361–78.
69. Livesley WJ, Jang KL. Toward an empirically based classification of personality disorder. J Personal Disord. 2000;14(2):137–51.
70. Sharp C, Fonagy P. Practitioner review: borderline personality disorder in adolescence—recent conceptualization, intervention, and implications for clinical practice. J Child Psychol Psychiatry. 2015;56(12):1266–88.
71. Richter J, Brunner R, Parzer P, Resch F, Stieltjes B, Henze R. Reduced cortical and subcortical volumes in female adolescents with borderline personality disorder. Psychiatry Res. 2014;221:179–86.

72. Driessen M, Herrmann J, Stahl K, et al. Magnetic resonance imaging volumes of hippocampus and the amygdala in women with borderline personality disorder and early traumatization. Arch Gen Psychiatry. 2000;57:1115–22.
73. Schmahl CG, Vermetten E, Elzinga BM, Douglas BJ. Magnetic resonance imaging volumes of the hippocampus and the amygdala volume in women with childhood abuse and borderline personality disorder. Psychiatry Res. 2003;122:193–8.
74. Tebartz van Elst L, Hesslinger B, Thiel T, Geiger E, Haegele K, Lemieux L, Lieb K, Bohus M, Hennig J, Ebert D. Frontolimbic brain abnormalities in patients with borderline personality disorder: a volumetric magnetic resonance imaging study. Biol Psychiatry. 2003;54:163–71.
75. Lyoo IK, Han MH, Cho DY. A brain MRI study in subjects with borderline personality disorder. J Affect Disord. 1998;50(2–3):235–43.
76. Hazlett EA, New AS, Newmark R, Haznedar MM, Lo JN, Speiser LJ, Chen AD, Mitropoulou V, Minzenberg M, Siever LJ, et al. Reduced anterior and posterior cingulate gray matter in borderline personality disorder. Biol Psychiatry. 2005;58:614–23.
77. Schmahl C, Bremner JD. Neuroimaging in borderline personality disorder. J Psychiatr Res. 2006;40:419–27.
78. Krause-Utz A, Elzinga BM, Oei NY, Paret C, Niedtfeld I, Spinhoven P, Bohus M, Schmahl C. Amygdala and dorsal anterior cingulate connectivity during an emotional working memory task in borderline personality disorder patients with interpersonal trauma history. Front Hum Neurosci. 2014;28(8):848.
79. Chanen AM, Velakoulis D, Carison K, Gaunson K, Wood SJ, Yuen HP, Yücel M, Jackson HJ, McGorry PD, Pantelis C. Orbitofrontal, amygdala and hippocampal volumes in teenagers with first-presentation borderline personality disorder. Psychiatr Res. 2008a;163:116–25.
80. Brunner R, Henze R, Parzer P, Kramer J, Feigl N, Lutz K, Essig M, Resch F, Stieltjes B. Reduced prefrontal and orbitofrontal gray matter in female adolescents with borderline personality disorder: is it disorder specific? NeuroImage. 2010;49:114–20.
81. Chanen AM, Jackson HJ, McCutcheon LK, et al. Early intervention for adolescents with borderline personality disorder using cognitive analytic therapy: randomised controlled trial. Br J Psychiatry. 2008b;193(6):477–84.
82. Goodman M, Hazlett EA, Avedon JB, Siever DR, Chu K-W, New AS. Anterior cingulate volume reduction in adolescents with borderline personality disorder and comorbid major depression. J Psychiatr Res. 2011;45:803–7.
83. Whittle S, Chanen AM, Fornito A, McGorry PD, Pantelis C, Yücel M. Anterior cingulate volume in adolescents with first-presentation borderline personality disorder. Psychiatry Res. 2009;172:155–60.
84. New AS, Carpenter DM, Perez-Rodriguez MM, Ripoll LH, Avedon J, Patil U, Hazlett EA, Goodman M. Developmental differences in diffusion tensor imaging parameters in borderline personality disorder. J Psychiatr Res. 2013;47:1101–9.
85. Maier-Hein KH, Brunner R, Lutz K, Henze R, Parzer P, Feigl N, Kramer J, Meinzer H-P, Resch F, Stieltjes B. Disorder-specific white matter alterations in adolescent borderline personality disorder. Biol Psychiatry. 2014;75:81–8.
86. Silbersweig D, Clarkin JF, Goldstein M, Kernberg OF, Tuescher O, Levy KN, Brendel G, Pan H, Beutel M, Pavony MT, et al. Failure of frontolimbic inhibitory function in the context of negative emotion in borderline personality disorder. Am J Psychiatry. 2007;164:1832–41.
87. Stoffers J, Vollm BA, Rucker G, Timmer A, Huband N, Lieb K. Pharmacological interventions for borderline personality disorder. Cochrane Database Syst Rev. 2010;16(6):CD005653.
88. Stoffers J, Vollm BA, Rucker G, Timmer A, Huband N, Lieb K. Psychological therapies for people with borderline personality disorder. Cochrane Database Syst Rev. 2012;8:CD005652.
89. Stoffers JM, Lieb K. Pharmacotherapy for borderline personality disorder—current evidence and recent trends. Curr Psychiatry Rep. 2015;17(1):534.
90. Oldham JM. Guideline watch. Practice guideline for the treatment of patients with borderline personality disorder. Arlington VA: American Psychiatric Association; 2005.
91. Linehan M. Cognitive behavior therapy of borderline personality disorder. New York, NY: Guilford; 1993.

92. Bateman AW, Fonagy P. Mentalization-based treatment of BPD. J Personal Disord. 2004;18(1):36–51.
93. Angus L, Gillies LA. Counseling the borderline client: an interpersonal approach. Can J Couns. 1994;28:69–82.
94. Markowitz JC, Skodol AE, Bleiberg K. Interpersonal psychotherapy for borderline personality disorder: possible mechanisms of change. J Clin Psychol. 2006;62:431–44.
95. Bellino S, Bozzatello P, De Grandi E, Bogetto F. Interpersonal psychotherapy: a model of intervention for borderline personality disorder. Riv Psichiatr. 2014;49(4):158–63.
96. Bozzatello P, Bellino S. Combined therapy with interpersonal psychotherapy adapted for borderline personality disorder: a two-years follow-up. Psychiatry Res. 2016;30(240):151–6.
97. Chanen AM, Thompson KN. Prescribing and borderline personality disorder. Aust Prescr. 2016;39(2):49–53.
98. Amminger GP, Chanen AM, Ohmann S, Klier CM, Mossaheb N, Bechdolf A, et al. Omega-3 fatty acid supplementation in adolescents with borderline personality disorder and ultra-high risk criteria for psychosis: a post hoc subgroup analysis of a double-blind, randomized controlled trial. Can J Psychiatry. 2013;58(7):402–8.
99. Ryle A, Kerr IB. Introducing cognitive analytic therapy: principles and practice. Chichester: Wiley; 2002.
100. Chanen AM, McCutcheon LK, Germano D, Nistico H, Jackson HJ, McGorry PD. The HYPE clinic: an early intervention service for borderline personality disorder. J Psychiatr Pract. 2009a;15(3):163–72.
101. Chanen AM, Jackson HJ, McCutcheon LK, Jovev M, Dudgeon P, Yuen HP, et al. Early intervention for adolescents with borderline personality disorder: quasi-experimental comparison with treatment as usual. Aust N Z J Psychiatry. 2009b;43(5):397–408.
102. Schuppert HM, Giesen-Bloo J, van Gemert TG, et al. Effectiveness of an emotion regulation group training for adolescents—a randomized controlled pilot study. Clin Psychol Psychother. 2009;16(6):467–78.
103. Blum N, St John D, Pfohl B, et al. Systems training for emotional predictability and problem solving (STEPPS) for outpatients with borderline personality disorder: a randomized controlled trial and 1-year follow-up. Am J Psychiatry. 2008;165(4):468–78.
104. Schuppert HM, Timmerman ME, Bloo J, et al. Emotion regulation training for adolescents with borderline personality disorder traits: a randomized controlled trial. J Am Acad Child Adolesc Psychiatry. 2012;51(12):1314–1323.e2.
105. Bateman A, Fonagy P. Mentalization based treatment for borderline personality disorder. World Psychiatry. 2010;9:11–5.
106. Rossouw TI, Fonagy P. Mentalization-based treatment for self-harm in adolescents: a randomized controlled trial. J Am Acad Child Adolesc Psychiatry. 2012;51(12): 1304–13.
107. Beck E, Bo S, Jørgensen MS, Gondan M, Poulsen S, Storebø OJ, Fjellerad Andersen C, Folmo E, Sharp C, Pedersen J, Simonsen E. Mentalization-based treatment in groups for adolescents with borderline personality disorder: a randomized controlled trial. J Child Psychol Psychiatr. 2020;61:594.
108. Mehlum L, Tørmoen AJ, Ramberg M, Haga E, Diep LM, Laberg S, Larsson BS, Stanley BH, Miller AL, Sund AM, Grøholt B. Dialectical behavior therapy for adolescents with repeated suicidal and self-harming behavior: a randomized trial. J Am Acad Child Adolesc Psychiatry. 2014;53(10):1082–91.
109. Mehlum L, Ramberg M, Tørmoen AJ, Haga E, Diep LM, Stanley BH, Miller AL, Sund AM, Grøholt B. Dialectical behavior therapy compared with enhanced usual care for adolescents with repeated suicidal and self-harming behavior: outcomes over a one-year follow-up. J Am Acad Child Adolesc Psychiatry. 2016;55(4):295–300.
110. Clarkin JF, Foelsch PA, Levy KN, Hull JW, Delaney JC, Kernberg OF. The development of a psychodynamic treatment for patients with borderline personality disorder: a preliminary study of behavioral change. J Personal Disord. 2001;15(6):487–95.

111. Chanen AM, McCutcheon LK. Personality disorder in adolescence: the diagnosis that dare not speak its name. Pers Ment Health. 2008;2(1):35–41.
112. Gunderson JG, Daversa MT, Grilo CM, McGlashan TH, Zanarini MC, Shea MT, Skodol AE, Yen S, Sanislow CA, Bender DS, Dyck IR, Morey LC, Stout RL. Predictors of 2-year outcome for patients with borderline personality disorder. Am J Psychiatry. 2006;163(5):822–6.
113. Winograd G, Cohen P, Chen H. Adolescent borderline symptoms in the community: prognosis for functioning over 20 years. J Child Psychol Psychiatry. 2008;49(9):933–41.
114. Newton-Howes G, Clark LA, Chanen A. Personality disorder across the life course. Lancet. 2015;385(9969):727–34.
115. Zanarini MC, Temesa CM, Frankenburg FR, Reich DB, Fitzmaurice GM. Description and prediction of time-to-attainment of excellent recovery for borderline patients followed prospectively for 20 years. Psychiatry Res. 2018;262:40–5.

Clinical Evaluation and Intervention of Emerging Psychosis: A Mentalization-Informed Perspective

7

Martin Debbané, George Salaminios, Jonas Weijers, Peter Fonagy, Eduardo Fonseca-Pedrero, and Marco Armando

M. Debbané (✉)
Faculty of Psychology and Educational Sciences, Developmental Clinical Psychology Research Unit, University of Geneva, Geneva, Switzerland

Research Department of Clinical, Educational and Health Psychology, University College London, London, UK

Developmental Imaging and Psychopathology, Department of Psychiatry, University of Geneva, Geneva, Switzerland
e-mail: Martin.Debbane@unige.ch

G. Salaminios
Research Department of Clinical, Educational and Health Psychology, University College London, London, UK

British Association for Counselling and Psychotherapy, Lutterworth, UK
e-mail: g.salaminios@ucl.ac.uk

J. Weijers
Rivierduinen Institute for Mental Health Care, Leiden, The Netherlands

Department of Psychiatry and Neuropsychology, School for Mental Health and Neuroscience, Maastricht University, Maastricht, The Netherlands

P. Fonagy
Research Department of Clinical, Educational and Health Psychology, University College London, London, UK
e-mail: p.fonagy@ucl.ac.uk

E. Fonseca-Pedrero
Departamento de Ciencias de la Educación, Universidad de La Rioja, La Rioja, Spain

Mental Health Networking Biomedical Research Centre (CIBERSAM), Oviedo, Spain

M. Armando
Developmental Imaging and Psychopathology, Department of Psychiatry, University of Geneva, Geneva, Switzerland

Service Universitaire de Psychiatrie de l'Enfant et de l'Adolescent, Centre Hospitalier Universitaire Vaudois (CHUV), Lausanne, Switzerland
e-mail: Marco.Armando@chuv.ch

P. Rocca, S. Bellino (eds.), *Psychosis and Personality Disorders*,
https://doi.org/10.1007/978-3-031-09058-5_7

Schizophrenia spectrum and other psychotic disorders (SSPDs) are currently conceptualized as disorders of neurodevelopment, where both genetic and environmental factors shape the propensity of individuals to experience alienating states of mind such as thought control delusions, auditory verbal hallucinations, feelings of persecution, and a sense of loss of agency over one's own being. While the concept of schizophrenia has been employed for more than a century [1], it is only recently that attention has been devoted to describing the slow and insidious developmental risk that precedes clinical states of psychosis, together with the various emergence patterns that characterize SSPDs. While this shift in clinical and scientific attention to the so-called premorbid and prodromal periods have fostered innovation in early clinical evaluation and intervention, the success of the first 20 years of clinical care before the onset of psychosis is mitigated [2]. Indeed, some trajectories toward SSPDs can be delayed or even avoided, but serious functional impairments prevail. For individuals who go on to experience SSPDs, symptomatic remission is often achieved through a combination of pharmacological and psychosocial treatment, yet functional remission in terms of role functioning, social integration, and self-management lags behind; this phenomenon is referred to as the symptom-disability gap [3]. In this chapter, we argue that one potentially fruitful way to address the challenges that preventive treatments in clinical disorders of psychosis (SSPDs) face, including the symptom-disability gap, is by integrating *mentalizing*, a developmentally acquired social cognitive function, to our understanding of emerging psychosis risk. We will first outline the evidence suggesting that mentalizing is a construct relevant to the emergence of and resilience against risk for psychosis. Within our developmental account of SSPDs, we frame mentalizing as a protective factor that may play a key role along the therapeutic pathway. In order to provide an illustration of the clinical continuum of psychosis, we include a clinical case description, the case of Dana, treated by two of the authors, with specific descriptions corresponding to the different periods of unfolding psychotic psychopathology. We will conclude with an overview of an evaluation and intervention paradigm informed by mentalization-based therapy (MBT) principles applied to emerging psychosis. MBT is an integrative therapeutic approach aiming to address distressing mental states through the process of mentalizing.

7.1 SSPDs and Mentalizing: Is There a Connection?

Mentalizing refers to the imaginative capacity required to interpret behavior, one's own and that of others, in terms of intentional mental states such as intentions, beliefs, desires, emotions, and the like [4]. Mentalizing mostly operates automatically, implicitly, and strongly impacts perception, attention, emotion regulation, memory, meaning-making, and behavior. As such, mentalizing would appear quite relevant to the manifestations of the three main classes of symptoms characteristic of SSPDs: (1) Positive symptoms, manifest through hallucinatory, and delusional experiences; (2) Negative symptoms, manifest through blunted affect, avolition, anhedonia, and social withdrawal; and (3) Disorganization symptoms, manifest through disorganization in thought, speech, and behavior. However, while mentalizing carries good face validity as causative factor to psychotic symptom manifestations, little evidence currently suggests that mentalizing is causally related to these clinical manifestations. As we have argued elsewhere, it would be premature to argue that mentalizing deficits increase the likelihood of SSPDs [5]. Currently, the picture is complex, as portrayed by the case of autism spectrum disorders (ASD): while ASD almost invariably involves severe mentalizing impairments, only 10–15% of cases go on to develop SSPDs [6]. In borderline personality disorder (BPD), also characterized by impairments of mentalizing, although only in context of emotional arousal, psychotic symptoms such as auditory verbal hallucinations are reported in up to 50% of individuals with the diagnosis of BPD [7]. From these correlational results, we can infer an association between psychotic symptoms and mentalizing impairments. But what is the nature of this association?

The best available answer to date is that the precise nature of the association(s) between SSPDs and mentalizing impairments remains elusive. As will become clearer below, our own working hypothesis takes a perspective grounded in salutogenesis: we hypothesize that mentalizing is a protective factor to psychopathology in general, and specifically in SSPDs, mentalizing protects the individual from the pathogenic effects of psychotic symptoms [5, 8]. As such, mentalizing may constitute one of the key therapeutic factors in SSPDs [9]. To date, the clearest instantiation of our hypothesis comes from the study of Emmanuel Peters and colleagues on a sample of adults with enduring psychotic symptoms [10]. In this study, the authors examined clinical, sociodemographic, and psychological characteristics in a group of individuals experiencing persistent psychotic symptoms (N total = 176), in comparison to a group of typical individuals without psychotic symptoms (N = 83). A key question stemming from our portraying of mentalizing as protective of psychopathology is to look for factors distinguishing psychotic symptoms requiring the need for care, versus psychotic symptoms not requiring care. Interestingly, this is exactly the question that Peters et al. examined in this study. A number of key psychological mechanisms were found to differentiate participants experiencing enduring symptoms but not needing care (N = 91) from those needing care (N = 82). Notably, a more negative self-image, less self-acceptance, and stronger negative core schemas characterized individuals needing care. Furthermore, participants not needing any care in relation to their persistent psychotic symptoms scored at the same level as typical controls on a number of variables. One result stood out, however, participants without need for care rated significantly higher on a measure of mindfulness, compared to both typical individuals without symptoms and individuals in need of care for their symptoms. Specifically, responding mindfully to negative thoughts and images was the only mechanism for which individuals not needing care outscored typical controls. How does this relate to our mentalization-informed hypothesis? We interpret these results as suggesting that while strong mentalizing, particularly self-mentalizing, does not protect from experiencing enduring psychotic symptoms, it can sustain a variety of beneficial effects [11], notably on self-image, core self-beliefs, and a capacity to mindfully respond to powerfully strong negative thoughts and images. It may be that an enhanced capacity to process negative thoughts and images actively defuses the psychopathological effect of enduring SSPD symptoms and sustain resilience in the context of ongoing symptomatology.

Although the exact dynamics between the different components of self-mentalizing still require further research and precision, the results from Peters et al. [10] with adult participants are also consistent with evidence gathered on developmental cohorts at enhanced risk to develop psychosis. In line with the focus of our chapter on the premorbid period and the clinical high-risk states for psychosis, we need to consider that mentalizing is itself a developmental capacity. A number of studies report associations between the quality of mentalizing in youths and their vulnerability to SSPDs. We will review the evidence of developmental associations between mentalizing and emerging risk for SSPDs below, while in parallel presenting a clinical vignette illustrating the developmental course from psychosis risk to the onset of psychosis. Our goal will be to integrate the developmental evidence suggesting both protective effects of increased mentalizing during adolescence, as well as potential links between developmental risk factors, mentalizing impairments, and increased psychosis proneness for the onset of SSPDs.

7.2 Risk and Resilience in SSPD: A Developmental Account

In line with contemporary clinical research on SSPDs [12], psychotic disorders are currently conceptualized as (neuro)developmental disorders. Importantly, the etiology of psychotic disorders most probably builds on a strong and significant genetic basis [13]. This does not mean that early environmental adversity does not come into play; on the contrary, many developmental studies are uncovering what Paul H. Meehl referred to as interactions between psychosocial stress and polygenetic potentiators [14]. Elsewhere, we have reviewed at least five neurobiological routes in which early adversity, developmental trauma, and attachment insecurity may each contribute to increase the risk for the onset of a psychotic disorder (for a review, see [5]). The interaction between the neurobiological routes and the psychological, interpersonal, and social risk factors entails a clinical consequence: a careful history of relationship patterns, stressful life events, and developmental trauma will assist in framing the context in which psychosis (risk) is evaluated, and how these interactions may impact different functional areas at different periods along the clinical continuum linked to SSPDs. Within this developmental context, four separate periods generally compose the clinical continuum of psychotic disorders (Fig. 7.1).

The four chronological periods can be distinguished in terms of the presence, severity, and functional impact of psychotic symptoms. The premorbid period encompasses the developmental interval, from conception to the emergence of subclinical to clinical symptoms of psychosis. This period is most relevant to study distal risk factors, such as familial, perinatal, early neurodevelopmental, and environmental factors during childhood and adolescence that confer elevated risk for future development of psychosis. Pediatric psychopathological manifestations can

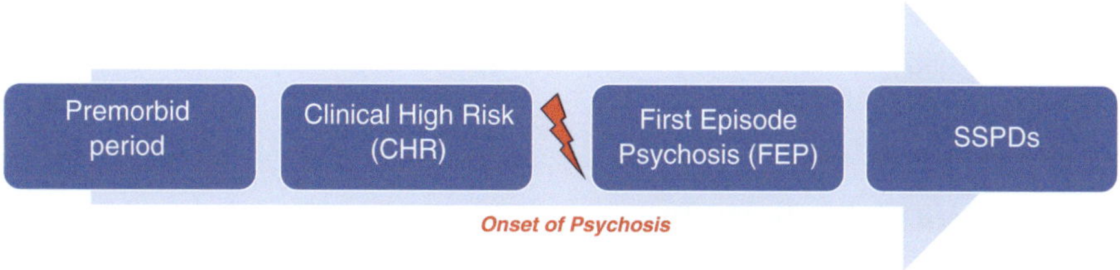

Fig. 7.1 Illustrating the clinical continuum associated with SSPDs (adapted from [15])

also predate the unfolding of SSPDs; mood and anxiety disorders, as well as neurodevelopmental disorders such as attention deficit with or without hyperactivity (ADHD), autism spectrum disorders (ASD), or other neurodevelopmental disorders can predate the onset of psychosis and augment risk to develop SSPDs [16].

It is estimated that approximately three-quarters of individuals who develop a psychotic disorder will first enter a period of clinical high-risk syndrome [17]. In the past two decades, two clinical paradigms have been proposed to evaluate clinical high-risk (CHR) of psychosis: the ultra-high risk (UHR) and the basic symptoms (BS) criteria [18, 19]. The UHR and BS criteria differ in phenomenology as well as in the way they are assessed clinically. The UHR paradigm evaluates the expression of attenuated positive symptoms, while BS are assessed on the basis of the individual's account of perceptive and cognitive disturbances subjectively signalling a shift in one's usual functioning [20, 21]. BS and UHR have been found to predict the onset of psychosis in approximately a quarter of individuals meeting the risk criteria [22].

The onset of psychosis is marked by the rise in frequency and severity of symptoms to a level meeting the diagnostic criteria of internationally recognized classification systems (ICD or DSM). It is often the case that while symptom severity and functional impact signal the presence of a clinical syndrome, the exact diagnoses require prolonged clinical observation. The term *First Episode Psychosis* (FEP) is a rather vague expression referring to the initial period where clinical psychosis is observed; it usually occurs between 15 and 30 years of age [23]. The clinical trajectory starting from psychosis onset depends upon a number of key factors, notably the level of premorbid functioning, the severity of negative and disorganization symptoms, and the duration of untreated psychosis [24]. These factors highlight the importance of early identification and prevention programs to reduce the morbidity associated with SSPDs [25]. The most prevalent clinical course after the initial diagnosis is one of recovery and relapse. Between 12 and 65% of individuals will progress within this category [26]. Up to a third of individuals may develop a more chronic disability, with a schizophrenic illness requiring substantial care [27].

Keeping in mind the different periods characterizing the subclinical to clinical continuum of psychosis expression, the clinical case presented below will provide an illustration of the developmental and clinical unfolding of SSPDs. Specifically, we will examine the four clinical periods along Dana's trajectory, from the premorbid period, through the CHR period leading to her FEP and clinical course with

SSPD. In parallel to the clinical vignette, we will provide the developmental research data suggesting a link between mentalizing and the psychosis continuum at each period of development.

7.2.1 Mentalizing in the Premorbid Period

The unfolding of psychotic psychopathology originates in the premorbid period, which is characterized by risk factors that are distally linked to the clinical expression of SSPDs. Part A of the clinical vignette describes the premorbid stage. The presence of risk factors encompassing familial risk, attachment issues, and experiences of trauma often interact within this period [5]. Early in her childhood, Dana describes what has been referred to as Psychotic-Like Experiences (PLEs: [28]).

Case Illustration of Dana (Part A): The Premorbid Period
Dana is the eldest of two children, born and raised in a number of different countries as the family moved around in relation to the father's work in international trade. Dana's father suffers from schizotypal personality disorder, and her mother was suspected to present borderline personality disorder. Dana was subject to intrafamilial sexual abuse as a child, and appears to have grown up in a familial environment characterized by physical and psychological neglect. She says her voice started during childhood. She remembers them as comforting voices that would "keep me company." They would appear irregularly, either when she was alone, or at night before she fell asleep. These voices would be relatively infrequent until mid-adolescence. The family sought psychiatric advice when Dana is between 9 and 11 years, a time during which her externalizing behavior was congruent with a conduct disorder diagnosis, and some sessions of individual and family therapy were attended at that time. Her average IQ was evaluated in the low mean average [29].

During development, PLEs present with similar phenomenology as positive symptoms of psychosis, yet do not meet the duration nor functional impact criteria to be considered above the clinical threshold. The seminal report from the Dunedin longitudinal study, where self-reported PLEs were assessed in 11-year olds and followed-up at age 26, initially suggested that such signs were predictors of early risk for late onset of SSPD [30]. However, when the predictive value of these early signs were tested through sensitivity and specificity analyses as the cohort participants reached the age of 38, such PLEs appeared to constitute relatively poor indicators of risk for transitioning to SSPD [31]. Other reports have suggested that early PLEs tend to disappear in more than 80% of cases [32]; however, they are predictive of a host of different psychopathological outcomes during adult age [33]. For those individuals with persistent PLEs, baseline emotional problems, together with behavioral problems and low cognitive functioning sustain the persistence of these manifestations along development [34]. Persistent PLEs carry a higher predictive value for psychotic disorders [35], especially when they are associated to high expression of schizotypy [32]. Schizotypy is a multidimensional personality trait that partly determines atypical patterns in neural functioning, affective dispositions, and information processing [36], which significantly determine the individual's relative risk to develop SSPDs [14].

Interestingly, several studies support the view that mentalizing capacity may moderate the expression of PLEs early during development. Bartels-Velthuis et al. [37] examined the potential influence of mentalizing capacity in the development of PLEs among children experiencing auditory hallucinations. The authors observed that better mentalizing capacities were associated with reduced persistence and development of PLEs over time [37]. Clemmensen and colleagues reported that children with below-average mentalizing scores were at an elevated risk of experiencing PLEs in comparison to children with above-average scores. These authors observed that PLEs in their samples were significantly associated with a hypermentalizing style, characterized by the over-attribution of intentions in others [38, 39]. These studies and others [40] illustrate the potential developmental interactions between maturing mentalizing capacities and early signs of psychosis risk such as PLEs.

Similarly, research on schizotypy expression has established developmental associations with specific mechanisms linked to self and other mentalizing during adolescence. A series of studies investigating reality monitoring mechanisms in typically developing youths highlighted associated between action monitoring and schizotypy [41, 42] as well as with internal speech monitoring [43]. In another study with a cohort of typically developing adolescents, levels of schizotypal expression of social anxiety and odd speech accounted for reduced usage of mental state information as measured by the Reflective Functioning Questionnaire [44]. Furthermore, poor usage of mental state information partially mediated the effects of social anxiety and odd speech on the level of thought problems in this sample [11]. In terms of self-mentalizing, the expression of schizotypy during adolescence appears to at least partly account for the propensity to experience self-face mirror illusions [45]. Using an experimental paradigm where teens are asked to continuously observe their specular image for 10 min under dimmed light conditions, participants reporting more positive and disorganized schizotypy experiences also reported more depersonalization-like illusions during the task, that is, experiencing the specular image as that of another person [46]. A recent developmental study administering the same mirror-gazing task in a sample of 216 participants aged between 7 and 30 years confirmed that the disorganization dimension of schizotypy played a role in augmenting the propensity to experience illusions all through development [47]. Furthermore, the positive schizotypy dimension best distinguished those experiencing depersonalization-like phenomena during the task to those reporting noninvasive illusions.

This ensemble of studies substantiates an association between pre-clinical signs of psychosis and mentalizing mechanisms, yet a suite of psychological processes appears to be involved in linking mentalizing and early signs of psychosis. Some studies focused on paradigms of theory of mind, which evaluate mental state processing of others, while more recent studies focus on mechanisms involved in mentalizing self. Research provides evidence linking both polarities of mentalizing to early signs of psychosis proneness in the premorbid period. Importantly, this suggests that mentalizing development may already influence the trajectory of risk for psychosis, while at the same time underlining that mentalizing impairments cannot be framed as a consequence of psychotic psychopathology. Along the clinical continuum of psychosis, there exists another opportunity to examine the role of mentalizing prior to the onset of psychosis, during the period of clinical high risk (CHR). Within this context, one key question to examine is whether the transition from an CHR state to the onset of a clinical disorder can be mitigated by mentalizing functions. We review the evidence surrounding this research question in the next section, in parallel to the continued presentation of Dana's clinical evolution within the CHR period.

7.2.2 Mentalizing in the CHR Period

The clinical high-risk period is characterized by either basic symptoms or attenuated psychotic symptoms that score above the CHR threshold, but under the clinical threshold for psychotic disorders. As of mid-adolescence, clinical evaluations of basic symptoms and ultra-high-risk symptoms are considered reliable, but this is less so during childhood and early adolescence [19].

Case Illustration of Dana (Part B): The High-Risk Stage
Around age 15, Dana's behavior is increasingly erratic; she presents with difficulties to concentrate, some disorganized speech and behavior, as well as strong opposition at home and in the school setting. Her peers tell her that she is weird, and she is victim of bullying during this period. When Dana drops out of school, she is eventually referred to a psychiatric service, where she receives a diagnosis of major depression, and attenuated psychotic symptoms. Her attenuated symptoms include voices that comment on her behavior, yet she appears to show some capacity to identify that these voices are not real, and that they are related to her psychological distress at school and with her parents.

Mentalizing processes are more generally part of social cognitive processes (e.g., ToM), which have been investigated by a number of different studies in light of their potential contribution to the transition between a CHR state and psychosis (see [48] for a review). Most studies fail to substantiate a link between social cognition deficits and the transition to a psychosis disorder. However, a more precise differentiation between the specific social cognitive functions assessed currently suggests that some basic mentalizing functions, such as the recognition of specific emotions and verbal theory of mind performances do carry predictive value for the transition into psychosis. One study suggests that poor performances in recognizing facial stimuli presenting either fear or neutral/ambiguous emotions were predictive of conversion to psychosis in subjects with CHR [49]. Another study found that verbal TOM predicted conversion to psychosis, although converting subjects also presented with lower general intelligence indices [50].

To the best of our knowledge, only one study involving individuals with CHR has specifically evaluated the predictive value of general mentalizing abilities, as opposed to component social cognitive processes, on the conversion to psychosis [40]. The strength of this study was to employ the most recognized measure of mentalizing, the interview-rated reflective functioning scale (RFS; Fonagy, Target [51]), which measures reflective functioning (RF) on the basis of the adult attachment interview [52]. The authors recruited 57 UHR and 53 non-UHR participants to investigate reflective functioning and transition to psychosis. The authors found that poor RF significantly related to Unusual Thought Content/Delusional Ideas, Suspiciousness/Persecutory Ideas, and Disorganized Communication subscales of the Structured Interview for Prodromal Symptoms (SIPS; [53]). Importantly, poor RF increased the likelihood of future transition to a psychotic disorder in the UHR group. This study adds to accumulating evidence that mentalizing may not only moderate the first signs of psychosis in the premorbid phase, but may also act as a protective factor in proximal periods of risk to transition toward clinical states of psychosis.

Clinical complexity within the CHR state cannot be reasonably represented without describing the important psychiatric comorbidity that most commonly accompanies CHR states. A recent study suggests that almost 40% of individuals meeting the UHR criteria also present with comorbid personality disorders [54], and another study suggests that general borderline personality pathology is present in approximately 25% of these individuals [55]. This suggests that clinicians providing treatment for these individuals should be trained in specialized PD psychotherapy models. Both mood and anxiety disorders further characterize the clinical picture of CHR; in a large sample of 509 individuals meeting the CHR criteria, three-quarters of individuals presented with an Axis I comorbid disorder [56]. An additional meta-analytical review reported baseline rates of mood (41%) and anxiety (15%) disorders in a sample of 1683 individuals with CHR for psychosis. The picture of comorbidity in CHR points to the importance of addressing emotional dysregulation at this stage of psychopathological progression, and it may be that a focus such as that proposed by mentalization-based-treatment may specifically mitigate risk for conversion by strengthening emotion regulation through more robust mentalizing in the individual and family, as we will describe below. Of note, the stability of persistence of CHR status varies between 28–78% within a 2–7.5 years' time frame, according to a recent meta-analysis of non-converting individuals with CHR [57]; importantly, their comorbid disorders yielded similar persistence within the same time interval. In line with these results, a secondary analysis of the Neurapro clinical trial found that in 202 individuals meeting the CHR criteria, poor outcome after 1 year (transition to psychosis, no remission or remission and relapse) was only predicted by general psychopathology. Together, these studies on prediction of conversion from CHR to psychosis, as well as long-term clinical outcomes of comorbid disorders underline the role of general (comorbid) psychopathology. These results further signify that a mentalization-informed approach to psychosis may be relevant: indeed, mentalization-based treatment is thought to reduce general psychopathology through enhancing the capacity to reflect on one's own experiences, as well as their experience of others. Furthermore, clinical evidence of mentalization-based treatment, although scarce, suggest it may assist in mitigating the poor functional outcomes commonly observed across the clinical continuum of psychosis [58–60]. In patients with SSPDs, MBT group intervention yielded beneficial effects on several measures of mentalizing, including ToM (hinting task), understanding of social causality (SCORS) and clinical self-insight (PANSS), and participants whose first psychotic episode had been less than 5 years prior seemed to profit more from the mentalization-focused group.

Together, studies on the premorbid and CHR periods sustain the hypothesis of a developmental association between mentalizing functions, progression of risk for psychosis, and the unfolding of unfavorable clinical and functional outcomes. Prediction models suggest that general psychopathology and functioning are predictive of unfavorable outcomes. In the next section, we describe the clinical approach informed by mentalization theory that may assist in evaluation and intervention during the early stages of SSPDs.

7.3 Clinical Implications of an Integrative Mentalization-Informed Perspective on SSPDs

Building on a developmental, mentalization-informed understanding of SSPDs, we wish to outline the clinical anchor points of our approach toward the process of evaluation and clinical intervention along the psychosis continuum. Figure 7.2 summarizes the main evaluation and intervention targets for each period along the continuum of expression of psychosis, from the premorbid to the potential chronic

CONTINUUM OF PSYCHOSIS

PERIODS / TARGETS	PRE-CLINICAL →	HIGH-RISK →	CLINICAL →	CHRONIC
EVALUATION	Familial / neurodevelopmental risk	Psychiatric comorbidity	Psychiatric comorbidity	Psychotic symptoms
	Attachment / Trauma	Basic Symptoms & Attenuated Psychotic Symptoms	Psychotic symptoms	Quality of life & Well-being
	(Social) Cognition	(Social) Cognition	(Social) Cognition	(Social) Cognition
	Risk screening indices	General and *interpersonal* functioning	General and *interpersonal* functioning	General and *interpersonal* functioning
INTERVENTION	Diet	Family Support	Family Support / Therapy	Family Support / Therapy
	Psychoeducation for risk groups	Psychosocial support	Psychosocial support	Psychosocial support
	Social skills & Emotion regulation	Psychotherapy	Psychotherapy	Psychotherapy (Group)
	Psychotherapy for Axis 1 disorders	*Psychopharmacology	Psychopharmacology	Psychopharmacology

*Psychopharmacology in the CHR period is currently a topic of debate (72)

Fig. 7.2 Illustrating the clinical continuum associated with SSPDs (adapted from [15]). *Psychopharmacology in the CHR period is currently a topic of debate [61]

periods. From the standpoint of mentalization-informed practice to evaluation, a few features stand out in comparison to evaluation as usual. First, the assessment of attachment patterns and developmental trauma is sensitively included in all evaluations. Their relevance is twofold. From an overall clinical perspective of psychopathology, it is now recognized that attachment patterns and trauma both contribute to treatment responses [62, 63], usually through their influence on the therapeutic alliance. They are also significantly linked to comorbidity and general psychopathology [64, 65], through their links with the development of attention and affect regulation mechanisms. Therefore, evaluating attachment patterns and trauma history will assist in preparing teams to sensitively engage clients into treatment. Second, from the clinical perspective of SSPDs specifically, attachment patterns are directly related to treatment engagement and response [66, 67], as is developmental trauma [68, 69]. The evaluation of attachment patterns will inform the assessment of functioning within the interpersonal domains; the practitioner may identify key protective relationships that may assist in treatment and clinical evolution. Knowledge on attachment anxiety, avoidance, and disorganization is thus quite useful when evaluating and treating SSPDs. Relatedly, expressed emotion in the interpersonal domain remains an area of clinical attention and intervention, as factors relating to affective arousal may trigger maladaptive attachment strategies, and influence the quality of mentalizing in all interpersonal relationships, especially within the family [70]. Indeed, a recent time-sensitive meta-analysis examining how expressed emotion components in the family relate to relapse in schizophrenia found that the level of critical comments and warmth independently influence the risk for relapse [71]. Finally, a mentalization-informed approach to evaluation will include specific assessments of cognitive and social-cognitive skills that can assist in tailoring treatment objectives, keeping a balance between scaffolding and challenging the learning process of (social) cognition and its application to real-life situations. Interestingly, a recent study involving a sample of 618 participants with SSPDs, reports that neurocognition prospectively predicts everyday life functioning, while avolition and social cognition predict interpersonal functioning [72]. If developmental differences in mentalizing exist between teens, young adults and adults, and inter-individual differences are present all along development, it is important to bear this in mind and adjust the level of interventions to levels contingent to the patient's capacities. Indeed individuals in their late teens and 20s are still developing their mentalizing skills [73], and thus require the appropriate support to scaffold their mentalizing of their own and other peoples' minds, which in turn will reinforce their emotion regulation capacities within the interpersonal domains.

In terms of intervention, the MBT framework has developed tools that can be appropriately adapted to periods of development, as well as different levels of psychosis expression. Following the evidence of early intervention trials [22], we note that dietary supplements in omega-3 fatty acid may be useful [74], although confirmatory evidence is still required; omega-3 fatty acid is thought to mitigate myelination vulnerability in at-risk populations, with potentially important roles in higher-order cognitive and regulation processes [75, 76]. In the premorbid period, psychoeducation and intervention during adolescence appear to sustain a number of key developmental processes, from mentalizing and emotion regulation [77] to identity and self-mentalizing processes [11, 60], especially in the context of affective turmoil in family and peer relationships. The MBT framework can be easily applied to the premorbid and CHR stages [78], supporting clients to reflect on their thoughts and feelings, as well as their perception of the thoughts, feelings, and intentions of others around them. As psychosis transitions from pre-clinical to clinical forms, multidisciplinary teams are required to address the needs of the patient and families. Adaptive Mentalization Based Integrative Treatment (AMBIT) may be useful to teams, especially in supporting multidisciplinary teams articulate their interventions when working with hard-to-reach clinical cases through case management models of care [79]. Indeed, all along the treatment trajectory, the MBT approach emphasizes the necessity to actively include family members in sustaining a reflective process around the client [80, 81]. Both reducing expressed emotion and facilitating communication patterns may strengthen psychological support between family members. For individuals suffering from chronic SSPDs, mentalization-based group therapy has shown to provide some clear benefits, both in terms of ameliorating mentalizing, as well as reducing social anxiety and hospitalization [58, 82, 83].

Continuing with Dana's case illustration, our goal is to illustrate how, the evaluation and treatment options evolve along the periods of progression of the illness and assist the attempts to mitigate the potential impact of psychotic psychopathology on mental health, role functioning, quality of life, and well-being.

Case Illustration of Dana (Part C): From CHR to Clinical Psychosis

During the month of December, just before her 16th birthday, Dana's psychotic symptoms flare and she begins the first of six hospitalizations during the following year. To cope with her symptoms, Dana describes patterns of social isolation, where only her mother can have psychological access to her. She additionally describes the importance of feeling physically connected to her mother by holding her hand, as if her mother's touch embodied her "lifeline" in those intense periods of suffering. At this point, the psychotic symptoms are fully clinical, in that they guide Dana's behavior and she cannot remain critical when she is experiencing these or when she attempts to reflect upon them. Her general functioning is evaluated as very low (GAF 35). She will undertake psychosocial treatment as well as antipsychotic medication.

In part C of Dana's clinical illustration, psychosis transitions from a clinical high-risk period to a first episode period. Could something have been done differently to delay or prevent this transition? This question has been at the center of early intervention in CHR over the past 20 years. A number of recent meta-analyses summarizing the potential impact of early intervention can be consulted on this topic [84]. Authors reviewing the evidence seem to converge on a number of key elements: (1) Intervening during the CHR stage is justified; (2) Approximately half of the cases at risk of transitioning can be either prevented or delayed; (3) The therapeutic impact on psychotic symptoms and social functioning is still very low, the comorbidity tends to persist; (4) The current evidence does not clearly point to superiority effects of any type of treatment, both psychological and antipsychotic treatment show effects. With this being said, the quality of the current evidence is relatively poor [2], notably due to limitations in sample size. Another research point worth reviewing, from our experience, is the type of coherence that can exist (or be lacking) in the network of care surrounding the patients. Many different types of professionals are involved in early intervention for clinical risk, and critical issues such as communication and continuity of care may lie in the way the different branches of care can come together from the perspective of the patient and family. Indeed, while delay or prevention of psychosis is a key target for treatment, the fact that general psychopathology and social functioning impairments do seem to persist suggests that these elements should be better integrated into preventive work. Interestingly, a number of more recent clinical trials specifically focus on social functioning [85], attempting to address the shortcomings of treatment, as well as the issues evoked in the first part of this chapter such as the symptom-disability gap.

Our own perspective on the issue would emphasize the need for a coherent multifaceted approach that can both address the issue of risk for psychosis, as well as general psychopathology, both occurring in the context of potentially impaired social cognitive function. As reviewed elsewhere [6], the different modalities of mentalization-based therapy (MBT) service delivery may be specifically useful to address the complexity and numerous challenges brought forth by emerging psychotic disorders [5]. It is unclear whether modular treatments represent therapeutically impactful solutions to current limitations in clinical interventions, as these modules can be difficult to integrate within general service delivery, and necessitate a level of engagement often difficult to sustain by patients and families [86]. Our experience is that a shared conceptual framework within multidisciplinary teams, which can be achieved through introductory training to MBT, will help build a common ground upon which articulation of interventions can broaden and facilitate the collaboration between the different professionals involved in the therapeutic journey: psychiatrists, clinical psychologists, mental health nurses, psychotherapists, educators, and other key workers that may be involved in any local service provision for emerging psychosis. Although research has yet to highlight this point, our experience suggests that being able to share a common framework of understanding around the patient and the family is one of the central aspects of treatment along the clinical continuum of psychosis. This does not mean that everyone is required to have psychotherapeutic expertise in one model, such as Cognitive Behavioral Therapy (CBT) or MBT, to be an effective treatment team. Rather, we suggest that the professional minds around the patient and family can have more impact through sharing a coherent and clear model of psychological suffering as a dynamic process, which involves psychological skills that are used to regulate difficult emotions, and that are required to think about one's own mind and that of others in ways that can foster psychological contact with a feeling of safety and trust. Mentalizing is about generating safety, trust, understanding, and collaboration between people [87]. Applied to SSPDs, a mentalizing-based approach seeks to provide an integrative framework where safety and trust when thinking about minds can be sufficiently and regularly experienced in order to be learned and used to mitigate the vigilance, distrust, and persecution that constitute the hallmark of mentalizing perturbations observed along the clinical continuum, and which inevitably induce anxiety, interpersonal avoidance, and social retreat [29].

Case Illustration of Dana (Part D): Trajectory with SSPD

After several attempts to engage in psychotherapy, Dana and her parents proposed an integrative treatment which included initially a semester of day hospital, concurrently with a weekly MBT psychotherapy session. In parallel, parent coaching was offered in an attempt to mitigate expressed emotion between the parents and the adolescent, a pattern that appeared to contribute to previous hospitalizations. Regular sessions with her psychiatrist were useful to monitor treatment adherence and pharmacological adaptations along the therapeutic journey, which lasted 3 years. Vocational training was also instrumental to assist Dana in pursuing attempts to find a place where she could both receive training and work. At the diagnostic level, schizophrenia was retained as principal diagnosis, together with comorbid depression and generalized anxiety.

The mentalization-based model was principally used in individual psychotherapy, which she found particularly important to defuse the anxiety around interpersonal relationships. MBT was also the basis for parent training, providing psychoeducation to identify the areas of affective arousal, cycles of loss of mentalizing within the family system. Mental health workers at the day hospital had received a short introductory training on MBT. Regular meetings with the care team were organized to share concerns and divide tasks when needed. At the termination of her therapeutic program, Dana had managed 18 months without any hospitalization, was in a professional curriculum and was involved in a romantic relationship for over a year. In her own words, Dana evoked the therapeutic journey with an increased capacity to hold herself in mind:

> I've gone through a lot in the past three years, hallucinations… hospitalizations… yeah gone through a lot and now… I am kind of proud of myself, I mean, I was at the very bottom of a hole.
>
> At age 15, I was in the abyss, totally, and now I am climbing the slope… I am climbing the ladder … I am climbing the ladder of life, and I am congratulating myself for this …

7.4 Conclusion

The reinforcement of mentalizing capacities is likely to have an effect on the regulation of thoughts and emotions, reducing the potential impact of psychosis on the individual's developmental trajectory. In Dana's case, the network of care was not able to delay or prevent transition to psychosis. Yet all the individuals involved in the program of care felt that important strides were achieved for Dana to secure a safe and caring relationship to herself, trust in professionals toward whom she could turn in times of need, as well as strengthen her regulation mechanisms to face everyday challenges and developmental tasks. Increased awareness of such "outcome measures," going beyond diagnostic issues and seeking to understand the complex interactions that take place to foster positive development in the face of psychosis is crucially needed to design future interventions.

In this chapter, we outlined the developmental associations between mentalizing and the emergence of SSPDs, suggesting that mentalizing may be framed as a protective factor that can reduce the pathogenic impact of psychosis, at different stages of psychopathological progression. A mentalization-informed approach will fail as a unique and miracle curative agent for psychosis, but will assist patients, family members, and professional's alike to maintain a focus on the mechanisms that can help cope with the affect-laden mental states that can be experienced as frightening, threatening and seemingly bizarre. More research is needed to better identify the mechanisms through which individuals with SSPDs can increase their capacity for self-mentalizing, to increase the impact of the quality of communication and the articulation of care on the success of treatment for SSPDs, and finally, understand the processes through which mentalization-informed treatment may benefit social and interpersonal functioning to decrease the symptom-disability gap.

References

1. Bleuler E. Dementia praecox or the group of schizophrenias (Zinkin J, Trans.). New York: International Universities Press; 1911/1950.
2. Bosnjak Kuharic D, Kekin I, Hew J, Rojnic Kuzman M, Puljak L. Interventions for prodromal stage of psychosis. Cochrane Database Syst Rev. 2019;2019(11):CD012236.
3. Birchwood M, Lester H, McCarthy L, Jones P, Fowler D, Amos T, et al. The UK national evaluation of the development and impact of Early Intervention Services (the National EDEN studies): study rationale, design and baseline characteristics. Early Interv Psychiatry. 2014;8(1):59–67.
4. Fonagy P, Gergely G, Jurist EL, Target M. Affect regulation, mentalization, and the development of the self. New York: Other Press; 2002.
5. Debbané M, Salaminios G, Luyten P, Badoud D, Armando M, Solida Tozzi A, et al. Attachment, neurobiology, and mentalizing along the psychosis continuum. Front Hum Neurosci. 2016;10:406.
6. De Giorgi R, De Crescenzo F, D'Alo GL, Rizzo Pesci N, Di Franco V, Sandini C, et al. Prevalence of non-affective psychoses in individuals with autism spectrum disorders: a systematic review. J Clin Med. 2019;8(9):1304.
7. Cavelti M, Thompson K, Chanen AM, Kaess M. Psychotic symptoms in borderline personality disorder: developmental aspects. Curr Opin Psychol. 2021;37:26–31.
8. Weijers JG, Ten Kate C, Debbané M, Bateman AW, de Jong S, Selten JP, et al. Mentalization and psychosis: a rationale for the use of mentalization theory to understand and treat non-affective psychotic disorder. J Contemp Psychother. 2020;50:223–32.
9. Debbané M, Bateman A. Psychosis. In: Bateman A, Fonagy P, editors. Handbook of mentalizing in mental health practice. 2nd ed. Washington, DC: American Psychiatric Association; 2019. p. 443–58.
10. Peters E, Ward T, Jackson M, Morgan C, Charalambides M, McGuire P, et al. Clinical, sociodemographic and psychological characteristics in individuals with persistent psychotic experiences with and without a "need for care". World Psychiatry. 2016;15(1):41–52.
11. Salaminios G, Debbané M. Sustaining the development of the self: mentalizing and recovery in the face of emerging psychosis. In: Hasson-Ohayion I, Lysaker PH, editors. The recovery of the self in psychosis. London: Routledge; 2021.

12. Rapoport JL, Addington AM, Frangou S, Psych MR. The neurodevelopmental model of schizophrenia: update 2005. Mol Psychiatry. 2005;10:434–49.
13. Lichtenstein P, Yip BH, Bjork C, Pawitan Y, Cannon TD, Sullivan PF, et al. Common genetic determinants of schizophrenia and bipolar disorder in Swedish families: a population-based study. Lancet. 2009;373(9659):234–9.
14. Debbané M, Barrantes-Vidal N. Schizotypy from a developmental perspective. Schizophr Bull. 2015;41(Suppl 2):S386–95.
15. Debbané M. Schizotypy: a developmental perspective. In: Mason O, Claridge G, editors. Schizotypy: new dimensions. London: Routledge; 2015.
16. Brasso C, Giordano B, Badino C, Bellino S, Bozzatello P, Montemagni C, et al. Primary psychosis: risk and protective factors and early detection of the onset. Diagnostics (Basel). 2021;11(11):2146.
17. Hafner H, Maurer K, Loffler W, an der Heiden W, Munk-Jorgensen P, Hambrecht M, et al. The ABC Schizophrenia Study: a preliminary overview of the results. Soc Psychiatry Psychiatr Epidemiol. 1998;33(8):380–6.
18. Michel C, Toffel E, Schmidt SJ, Eliez S, Armando M, Solida-Tozzi A, et al. Détection et traitement précoce des sujets à haut risque clinique de psychose: définitions et recommandations. L'Encéphale. 2017;43(3):292–7.
19. Schultze-Lutter F, Michel C, Schmidt SJ, Schimmelmann BG, Maric NP, Salokangas RK, et al. EPA guidance on the early detection of clinical high risk states of psychoses. Eur Psychiatry. 2015;30(3):405–16.
20. Schultze-Lutter F. Subjective symptoms of schizophrenia in research and the clinic: the basic symptom concept. Schizophr Bull. 2009;35(1):5–8.
21. Schultze-Lutter F, Debbane M, Theodoridou A, Wood SJ, Raballo A, Michel C, et al. Revisiting the basic symptom concept: toward translating risk symptoms for psychosis into neurobiological targets. Front Psychiatry. 2016;7:9.
22. Catalan A, Salazar de Pablo G, Vaquerizo Serrano J, Mosillo P, Baldwin H, Fernandez-Rivas A, et al. Annual research review: prevention of psychosis in adolescents—systematic review and meta-analysis of advances in detection, prognosis and intervention. J Child Psychol Psychiatry. 2021;62(5):657–73.
23. Breitborde NJ, Srihari VH, Woods SW. Review of the operational definition for first-episode psychosis. Early Interv Psychiatry. 2009;3(4):259–65.
24. Penttila M, Jaaskelainen E, Hirvonen N, Isohanni M, Miettunen J. Duration of untreated psychosis as predictor of long-term outcome in schizophrenia: systematic review and meta-analysis. Br J Psychiatry. 2014;205(2):88–94.
25. Davies C, Cipriani A, Ioannidis JPA, Radua J, Stahl D, Provenzani U, et al. Lack of evidence to favor specific preventive interventions in psychosis: a network meta-analysis. World Psychiatry. 2018;17(2):196–209.
26. Alvarez-Jimenez M, Gleeson JF, Henry LP, Harrigan SM, Harris MG, Killackey E, et al. Road to full recovery: longitudinal relationship between symptomatic remission and psychosocial recovery in first-episode psychosis over 7.5 years. Psychol Med. 2012;42(3):595–606.
27. AlAqeel B, Margolese HC. Remission in schizophrenia: critical and systematic review. Harv Rev Psychiatry. 2012;20(6):281–97.
28. Fonseca Pedrero E, Debbane M. Schizotypal traits and psychotic-like experiences during adolescence: an update. Psicothema. 2017;29(1):5–17.
29. Salaminios G, Morosan L, Toffel E, Tanzer M, Eliez S, Badoud D, et al. Associations between schizotypal personality features, mentalizing difficulties and thought problems in a sample of community adolescents. Early Interv Psychiatry. 2020;15(3):705–15.
30. Poulton R, Caspi A, Moffitt TE, Cannon M, Murray R, Harrington H. Children's self-reported psychotic symptoms and adult schizophreniform disorder: a 15-year longitudinal study. Arch Gen Psychiatry. 2000;57(11):1053–8.
31. Reichenberg A, Caspi A, Harrington H, Houts R, Keefe RS, Murray RM, et al. Static and dynamic cognitive deficits in childhood preceding adult schizophrenia: a 30-year study. Am J Psychiatry. 2010;167(2):160–9.

32. Debbané M, Eliez S, Badoud D, Conus P, Fluckiger R, Schultze-Lutter F. Developing psychosis and its risk States through the lens of schizotypy. Schizophr Bull. 2015;41(Suppl 2):S396–407.
33. Polari A, Yuen HP, Amminger P, Berger G, Chen E, deHaan L, et al. Prediction of clinical outcomes beyond psychosis in the ultra-high risk for psychosis population. Early Interv Psychiatry. 2021;15(3):642–51.
34. Steenkamp LR, Tiemeier H, Blanken LME, Hillegers MHJ, Kushner SA, Bolhuis K. Predicting persistence of hallucinations from childhood to adolescence. Br J Psychiatry. 2021;219(6):670–7.
35. Dominguez MD, Wichers M, Lieb R, Wittchen HU, van Os J. Evidence that onset of clinical psychosis is an outcome of progressively more persistent subclinical psychotic experiences: an 8-year cohort study. Schizophr Bull. 2011;37(1):84–93.
36. Lenzenweger MF. Schizotypy and schizophrenia: the view from experimental psychology. New York: The Guilford Press; 2010.
37. Bartels-Velthuis AA, Blijd-Hoogewys EM, van Os J. Better theory-of-mind skills in children hearing voices mitigate the risk of secondary delusion formation. Acta Psychiatr Scand. 2011;124(3):193–7.
38. Clemmensen L, van Os J, Drukker M, Munkholm A, Rimvall MK, Vaever M, et al. Psychotic experiences and hyper-theory-of-mind in preadolescence—a birth cohort study. Psychol Med. 2016;46(1):87–101.
39. Clemmensen L, van Os J, Skovgaard AM, Vaever M, Blijd-Hoogewys EMA, Bartels-Velthuis AA, et al. Hyper-theory-of-mind in children with psychotic experiences. PLoS One. 2014;9(11):e113082.
40. Boldrini T, Pontillo M, Tanzilli A, Giovanardi G, Di Cicilia G, Salcuni S, et al. An attachment perspective on the risk for psychosis: clinical correlates and the predictive value of attachment patterns and mentalization. Schizophr Res. 2020;222:209–17.
41. Debbané M, Van der Linden M, Gex-Fabry M, Eliez S. Cognitive and emotional associations to positive schizotypy during adolescence. J Child Psychol Psychiatry. 2009;50(3):326–34.
42. Dahoun T, Eliez S, Chen F, Badoud D, Schneider M, Laroi F, et al. Action simulation in hallucination-prone adolescents. Front Hum Neurosci. 2013;7:329.
43. Salaminios G, Morosan L, Toffel E, Tanzer M, Eliez S, Debbane M. Self-Monitoring for speech and its links to age, cognitive effort, schizotypal trait expression and impulsivity during adolescence. Cogn Neuropsychiatry. 2020;25(3):215–30.
44. Badoud D, Luyten P, Fonseca-Pedrero E, Eliez S, Fonagy P, Debbane M. The French version of the reflective functioning questionnaire: validity data for adolescents and adults and its association with non-suicidal self-injury. PLoS One. 2015;10(12):e0145892.
45. Fonseca-Pedrero E, Badoud D, Antico L, Caputo GB, Eliez S, Schwartz S, et al. Strange-face-in-the-mirror illusion and schizotypy during adolescence. Schizophr Bull. 2015;41(Suppl 2):S475–82.
46. Derome M, Fonseca-Pedrero E, Badoud D, Morosan L, Van De Ville D, Lazeyras F, et al. Resting-state networks of adolescents experiencing depersonalization-like illusions: cross-sectional and longitudinal findings. Schizophr Bull. 2018;44:S501–S11.
47. Derome M, Fonseca-Pedrero E, Caputo GB, Debbane M. A developmental study of mirror-gazing-induced anomalous self-experiences and self-reported schizotypy from 7 to 28 years of age. Psychopathology. 2021;55(1):49–61.
48. van Donkersgoed RJM, Wunderink L, Nieboer R, Aleman A, Pijnenborg GHM. Social cognition in individuals at ultra-high risk for psychosis: a meta-analysis. PLoS One. 2015;10(10):e0141075.
49. Allott KA, Schafer MR, Thompson A, Nelson B, Bendall S, Bartholomeusz CF, et al. Emotion recognition as a predictor of transition to a psychotic disorder in ultra-high risk participants. Schizophr Res. 2014;153(1–3):25–31.
50. Kim HS, Shin NY, Jang JH, Kim E, Shim G, Park HY, et al. Social cognition and neurocognition as predictors of conversion to psychosis in individuals at ultra-high risk. Schizophr Res. 2011;130(1–3):170–5.

51. Fonagy P, Target M, Steele H, Steele M. Reflective functioning scale manual. Unpublished manuscript, London. 1998.
52. George C, Kaplan N, Main M. The Berkeley adult attachment interview. Unpublished manuscript, Berkeley, CA. 1996.
53. McGlashan T. Structured interview for prodromal syndromes (SIPS). University Y, editor. New Haven. 2001.
54. Boldrini T, Tanzilli A, Pontillo M, Chirumbolo A, Vicari S, Lingiardi V. Comorbid personality disorders in individuals with an at-risk mental state for psychosis: a meta-analytic review. Front Psychiatry. 2019;10:429.
55. Ryan J, Graham A, Nelson B, Yung A. Borderline personality pathology in young people at ultra high risk of developing a psychotic disorder. Early Interv Psychiatry. 2017;11(3):208–14.
56. Fusar-Poli P, Nelson B, Valmaggia L, Yung AR, McGuire PK. Comorbid depressive and anxiety disorders in 509 individuals with an at-risk mental state: impact on psychopathology and transition to psychosis. Schizophr Bull. 2014;40(1):120–31.
57. Beck K, Andreou C, Studerus E, Heitz U, Ittig S, Leanza L, et al. Clinical and functional long-term outcome of patients at clinical high risk (CHR) for psychosis without transition to psychosis: a systematic review. Schizophr Res. 2019;210:39–47.
58. Weijers J, Ten Kate C, Viechtbauer W, Rampaart LJA, Eurelings EHM, Selten JP. Mentalization-based treatment for psychotic disorder: a rater-blinded, multi-center, randomized controlled trial. Psychol Med. 2020;51:1–10.
59. Lana F, Marcos S, Mollà L, Vilar A, Pérez V, Romero M, et al. Mentalization based group psychotherapy for psychosis: a pilot study to assess safety, acceptance and subjective efficacy. Int J Psychol Psychoanal. 2015;1(1):1–6.
60. Debbané M, Benmiloud J, Salaminios G, Solida-Tozzi A, Armando M, Fonagy P, et al. Mentalization-based treatment in clinical high-risk for psychosis: a rationale and clinical illustration. J Contemp Psychother. 2016;46(4):217–25.
61. Raballo A, Poletti M. Overlooking the transition elephant in the ultra-high-risk room: are we missing functional equivalents of transition to psychosis? Psychol Med. 2022;52(1):184–7.
62. Reis S, Grenyer BFS. Fearful attachment, working alliance and treatment response for individuals with major depression. Clin Psychol Psychot. 2004;11(6):414–24.
63. Bernecker SL, Levy KN, Ellison WD. A meta-analysis of the relation between patient adult attachment style and the working alliance. Psychother Res. 2014;24(1):12–24.
64. Groh AM, Roisman GI, van Ijzendoorn MH, Bakermans-Kranenburg MJ, Fearon RP. The significance of insecure and disorganized attachment for children's internalizing symptoms: a meta-analytic study. Child Dev. 2012;83(2):591–610.
65. Cerda M, Sagdeo A, Johnson J, Galea S. Genetic and environmental influences on psychiatric comorbidity: a systematic review. J Affect Disord. 2010;126(1–2):14–38.
66. Quijada Y, Tizon JL, Artigue J, Kwapil TR, Barrantes-Vidal N. Attachment style predicts 6-month improvement in psychoticism in persons with at-risk mental states for psychosis. Early Interv Psychiatry. 2012;6(4):442–9.
67. Quijada Y, Kwapil TR, Tizon J, Sheinbaum T, Barrantes-Vidal N. Impact of attachment style on the 1-year outcome of persons with an at-risk mental state for psychosis. Psychiatry Res. 2015;228(3):849–56.
68. Read J, van Os J, Morrison AP, Ross CA. Childhood trauma, psychosis and schizophrenia: a literature review with theoretical and clinical implications. Acta Psychiatr Scand. 2005;112(5):330–50.
69. Gumley AI, Taylor HE, Schwannauer M, MacBeth A. A systematic review of attachment and psychosis: measurement, construct validity and outcomes. Acta Psychiatr Scand. 2014;129(4):257–74.
70. Asen E, Fonagy P. Mentalizing family violence part 1: conceptual framework. Fam Process. 2017;56(1):6–21.
71. Ma CF, Chan SKW, Chung YL, Ng SM, Hui CLM, Suen YN, et al. The predictive power of expressed emotion and its components in relapse of schizophrenia: a meta-analysis and meta-regression. Psychol Med. 2021;51(3):365–75.

72. Mucci A, Galderisi S, Gibertoni D, Rossi A, Rocca P, Bertolino A, et al. Factors associated with real-life functioning in persons with schizophrenia in a 4-year follow-up study of the Italian network for research on psychoses. JAMA Psychiatry. 2021;78(5):550–9.
73. Badoud D, Speranza M, Debbané M. Vers un modèle du développement de la mentalisation à l'adolescence – Towards a developmental model of the mentalization dimensions during adolescence. Rev Qué Psychol. 2016:49–68. https://doi.org/10.3917/dbu.debba.2018.01.0239.
74. Amminger GP, Schafer MR, Papageorgiou K, Klier CM, Cotton SM, Harrigan SM, et al. Long-chain omega-3 fatty acids for indicated prevention of psychotic disorders: a randomized, placebo-controlled trial. Arch Gen Psychiatry. 2010;67(2):146–54.
75. Cutuli D, Pagani M, Caporali P, Galbusera A, Laricchiuta D, Foti F, et al. Effects of omega-3 fatty acid supplementation on cognitive functions and neural substrates: a voxel-based morphometry study in aged mice. Front Aging Neurosci. 2016;8:38.
76. Vijayakumar N, Bartholomeusz C, Whitford T, Hermens DF, Nelson B, Rice S, et al. White matter integrity in individuals at ultra-high risk for psychosis: a systematic review and discussion of the role of polyunsaturated fatty acids. BMC Psychiatry. 2016;16:287.
77. Rossouw TI, Fonagy P. Mentalization-based treatment for self-harm in adolescents: a randomized controlled trial. J Am Acad Child Adolesc Psychiatry. 2012;51(12):1304–13.e3.
78. Debbané M, Toffel E. Mentalizing through the early stages of the psychosis continuum. In: Pereira JG, de Almeida Gonçalves J, Bizzari V, editors. The neurobiology-psychotherapy-pharmacology intervention triangle. Wilmington: Vernon Press; 2019. p. 141–60.
79. Bevington D, Fuggle P, Fonagy P. Applying attachment theory to effective practice with hard-to-reach youth: the AMBIT approach. Attach Hum Dev. 2015;17(2):157–74.
80. Claxton M, Onwumere J, Fornells-Ambrojo M. Do family interventions improve outcomes in early psychosis? A systematic review and meta-analysis. Front Psychol. 2017;8:371.
81. Okpokoro U, Sampson S. Brief family intervention for schizophrenia. Schizophr Bull. 2014;40(3):497–8.
82. Weijers J. Mentalizing psychosis: trying to understand the un-understandable. Maastricht: Maastricht University; 2020.
83. Weijers J, Ten Kate C, Eurelings-Bontekoe E, Viechtbauer W, Rampaart R, Bateman A, et al. Mentalization-based treatment for psychotic disorder: protocol of a randomized controlled trial. BMC Psychiatry. 2016;16:191.
84. Mei C, van der Gaag M, Nelson B, Smit F, Yuen HP, Berger M, et al. Preventive interventions for individuals at ultra high risk for psychosis: an updated and extended meta-analysis. Clin Psychol Rev. 2021;86:102005.
85. Friedman-Yakoobian MS, Parrish EM, Eack SM, Keshavan MS. Neurocognitive and social cognitive training for youth at clinical high risk (CHR) for psychosis: a randomized controlled feasibility trial. Schizophr Res. 2020;243:302–6.
86. Glenthoj LB, Mariegaard LS, Fagerlund B, Jepsen JRM, Kristensen TD, Wenneberg C, et al. Cognitive remediation plus standard treatment versus standard treatment alone for individuals at ultra-high risk of developing psychosis: results of the FOCUS randomised clinical trial. Schizophr Res. 2020;224:151–8.
87. Luyten P, Campbell C, Allison E, Fonagy P. The mentalizing approach to psychopathology: state of the art and future directions. Annu Rev Clin Psychol. 2020;16:297–325.

Personality Disorders and Suicidality 8

Marco Sarchiapone and Patrizia Zeppegno

8.1 Introduction

According to DSM 5, personality disorders are characterized by a pervasive and stable pattern of "inner experience and behavior," present at least from adolescence, which is deviant from a person's cultural norms [1, 2]. These patterns of inner experience and behavior tend to be inflexible and emerge across abroad range of situations. Essential features of personality disorders are severe impairment in personality functioning, as well as inself functioning (identity or self-direction) and interpersonal functioning (empathy or intimacy). Other criteria are that these impairments in personality functioning and the individual's personality trait expression are relatively stable across time and consistent across situations; they are not better understood as normative for the individual's developmental stage or sociocultural environment and are not only due to the direct physiological and psychological effects of a substance (e.g., alcohol, drugs, and medications) or a general medical condition (e.g., severe head trauma) (DSM-5 Criteria-Revised June 2011). The impact of personality disorders reverberates on patients' interpersonal relationships, as well as on their social and occupational functioning. Management of personality disorders is often a hard challenge for psychiatric services, due to severity of illness, chronic clinical course, and issues regarding high-risk behaviors such as substance abuse, self-harm, non-suicidal self-injuries, suicide attempts, and suicidality [3]. The current literature is much more focused on Axis I disorders and their correlation

M. Sarchiapone
Department of Medicine and Health Sciences, University of Molise, Campobasso, Italy

P. Zeppegno (✉)
Department of Translational Medicine, Università degli Studi del Piemonte Orientale, Scuola di Medicina, Novara, Italy

Psychiatry Ward, Azienda Ospedaliero Universitaria Maggiore della Carità, Novara, Piemonte, Italy
e-mail: patrizia.zeppegno@med.uniupo.it

P. Rocca, S. Bellino (eds.), *Psychosis and Personality Disorders*,
https://doi.org/10.1007/978-3-031-09058-5_8

with suicide, rather than on Axis II disorders. Findings show a correlation between suicide with major depression (85.2% of cases), bipolar disorder (7.4%), and schizophrenia (3.3%) [4]. Nonetheless, personality disorders are a considerable risk factor for suicidal behavior predicting completed suicide in follow-up [5]. More specifically, especially those personality disorders (like Borderline Personality disorder and other Cluster B personality disorders) which are associated with features like impulsiveness, aggression, depression, and affective dysregulation are often related to suicidality and suicidal behavior [6].

Indeed, suicidal behaviors are not limited to suicide but encompass a wide range of behaviors, including suicidal ideation, non-suicidal self-injury, suicide attempt, and non-fatal suicidal behavior; all of these should be considered as warning signs and possible predictors of suicide [7–10]. Notably, not only suicide is a common feature among individuals with personality disorders, but overall suicidal behaviors, as described above, are frequent in this population.

Suicide is a complex phenomenon that does not only involve psychiatric patients as it deeply concerns human beings and hence the entire population. According to the World Health Organization (WHO), close to 800,000 people die due to suicide every year: this indicates an annual global age-standardized suicide rate of 10.5 per 100,000 population [11]. Suicide is also the second leading cause of death in young (15–29 years) people [12]. According to current literature [13], suicide is defined as death caused by self directed injurious behavior with an intent to die as a result of the behavior; a suicide attempt is defined as a non-fatal, self-directed, potentially injurious behavior with an intent to die as a result of the behavior even if the behavior does not result in injury. A failed suicide is intended as a self-harm behavior with the intent to die where death not occurs by reasons that do not depend on the attempter's will, and suicidal ideation is defined as thinking about, considering, or planning suicide. Other related behaviors could include non-suicidal self-injury where the intent of hurting oneself is not linked with the intent to die.

The scientific literature and epidemiological data suggest that suicide occurs at least 10 times more frequently in psychiatric patients than in the general population [14]. According to worldwide data, psychiatric patients at highest risk for suicide include those suffering from depression (30%), followed by those with substance use-related disorders (18%), schizophrenia (14%), and personality disorders (13%) [15].

It is widely acknowledged by the current literature that a history of attempted suicide is the most important predictive factor for completed suicide, and indeed about 25% of suicide attempters have shown suicidal behaviors in the past year [5, 16]. Furthermore, the relationship between non-suicidal self-injury and deliberate-self harm and suicide has been discussed and debated in the literature [5, 16], and as such behaviors have a high frequency in personality disorders, these should be considered high-risk diagnoses.

It should be also underscored that "Recurrent suicidal behavior, gestures, or threats, or self-mutilating behavior" is one of the diagnostic criteria for Borderline Personality disorder, and that, overall, personality disorders, especially cluster B ones, may display several psychological features which have been reported in association with suicidal behavior (e.g., impulsivity, emotional instability, and feelings of emptiness). Indeed, most results available in the current scientific literature about personality disorders and suicidality deal with borderline personality disorder. Findings witness that suicide attempters display higher aggression levels than non-attempters [17] and support the hypothesis that patients showing affective dysregulation might be more likely to display self-aggression (i.e., suicide attempts) when facing negative emotions such as guilt, anger, or self-hatred. Nonetheless, this kind of dysregulation is not only a feature of borderline personality disorder, but it is also shared by narcissistic personality disorders, where emotional dysregulation and impulsive aggression associated with failure to meet self and other's expectations might result in interpersonal hostile or aggressive behaviors [18].

8.1.1 Personality Disorders and Suicidality

Personality disorders have been described as a risk factor for suicidal behavior, predicting completed suicide at 10–15 years follow-up. With more detail, compared to other psychiatric disorders and to individuals with no history of psychiatric disorders, personality disorders showed a fourfold and 20-fold increase in suicide risk, respectively [19]. In a large number of suicide attempters and suicide victims, it was found at least one personality disorder [20]. Other data from long-term follow-up studies show a percentage of complete suicide ranging from 3 to 9% in borderline personality disorder patients [21, 22]. In an overview of the literature, some authors found that patients with borderline personality disorder represent from 9 to 33% of all suicides [23, 24]; this variability may suggest critical issues concerning diagnosis.

As already underscored, borderline appears to be the most studied personality disorder as risk factor for suicide; nonetheless, other personality disorders were found to be linked to suicide, though with a weaker association.

Cluster A personality disorders do not appear to be significant risk factors for suicide. Nonetheless, in a study where psychological autopsy was performed on suicidal Israeli males during military service, the most common personality disorders were schizoid (37.2%) and narcissistic personality disorder (23.3%) [25]. Also, a more recent study suggested an association between symptoms of schizoid personality disorders (such as interpersonal difficulties and low levels of emotional expressions) and suicide [26].

Regarding Cluster B personality disorders, the relationship between a narcissistic personality disorder and a higher risk of dying by suicide [27] has been supported, as well as an association between less impulsivity but more lethality of attempts in this group of patients [28]. This relationship could be explained considering narcissistic traits like pride or amplified response to social failure. As far as antisocial personality disorder is concerned, a relationship with suicide attempt can be found, usually with a drug overdose and in order to obtain a secondary gain; on the other hand, the rate of completed suicide is significantly lower compared to other personality disorders, likely due to a low lethality of attempts [29].

Regarding substance abuse and alcoholism, studies found that the comorbid use of alcohol or substances with borderline personality disorder raised the perception of a higher risk of suicidal behavior on behalf of patients [30]. Briefly, the severity of suicidal risk in borderline personality disorder, according to longitudinal studies is related to the following: psychiatric comorbidity, especially with depressive disorder; alcohol and substance abuse; impulsivity, aggression, and hostility; repeated attempts; antisocial traits; severity of borderline personality disorder [31, 32]. All these high-risk factors may be triggered by stressful life events like affective and sentimental difficulties (e.g., separation from a partner, end of a relationship) or life events that imply a change (problems with relatives, work issues, or discharge) [33, 34]. It is likely that stressful life events may be particularly problematic for patients with a personality disorder, as they may have poor coping skills to face them.

Last, Cluster C personality disorders showed no strong association with suicide in studies after controlling for Axis I disorders [35], while the association between Cluster A and Cluster B personality disorders and suicide attempts seemed to maintain significance even after controlling for depression and its severity [36].

Overall, guidelines underscore the importance of appropriately diagnosing and addressing disorders underlying suicidal behaviors, especially depression, anxiety, substance abuse, and personality disorders, in order to achieve successful prevention of suicidality [37].

8.1.1.1 Developmental Trajectories of Self-injury Behaviors and Borderline Personality Disorders

Studies in the context of suicide prevention programs targeting adolescent populations have yielded some interesting results. Self-injurious behavior and risk-taking behaviors are associated with adolescent borderline personality disorder (BPD), although their developmental trajectories in predicting BPD have not been fully understood. In the context of the Saving and Empowering Young Lives in Europe, data from 506 adolescents from Germany were analyzed, highlighting the importance of some facets of risk-taking behaviors in the development of adolescent BPD. Among these facets, the most relevant ones, which highest OR, were self-injurious behaviors and alcohol termination [38].

The investigation of direct self-injurious behavior (D-SIB) in the same sample of adolescents revealed that onset and maintenance of D-SIB between baseline and 1-year follow-up were associated with an increased risk for suicidal thoughts and behavior at 2-years follow-up. On the other hand, interestingly, D-SIB cessation before the 1-year follow-up reduced later risk for suicidal thoughts and behavior, which became comparable to those with no lifetime history of D-SIB [39].

In this cohort of adolescents, the developmental trajectories of self-injurious behavior (SIB), suicidal behavior (SB), and substance misuse (SM) and their association with BPD traits were investigated as well. A high degree of overlap (80–90%) was found among the high-risk trajectories for these three behaviors (SIB, SB, and SM), and was significantly associated with elevated levels of BPD pathology [40].

The possible role of trauma has been suggested as well. The association between childhood trauma and aggression was investigated in two distinct samples of Italian and French suicide attempters, for a total of 587 subjects with different psychiatric diagnoses (DSM-IV-TR criteria). Patients were assessed with the Brown-Goodwin Assessment for Lifetime History of Aggression (BGLHA) and the Childhood Trauma Questionnaire (CTQ). In both samples of Italian and French suicide attempters, significant correlations were found between childhood trauma and aggression [41].

8.1.1.2 Temperament and Character Correlates of Personality and Suicidality

Considering that suicide occurs also in people which are not diagnosed with a major psychiatric disease, understanding which personality features are related to suicidality is a very important research topic.

Several studies have investigated the temperamental and emotional correlates of personality and suicidality, which go beyond the diagnosis of a given psychiatric disorder and of a specific personality disorder. Currently, a valid reference model for the understanding of suicidal behavior is the stress-diathesis one. A diathesis is commonly conceptualized as a predispositional factor, or a set of factors, which could lead to a pathological state. This could include biological, genetic, but also cognitive and social factors. This model, which has a long history in medicine, postulates that suicide results from an interaction between state-dependent (environmental) stressors and a trait-like diathesis or susceptibility to suicidal behavior, independent of psychiatric disorders. In relation to this model, a high vulnerability to stress, or an exaggerated response to below-threshold stimuli could elicitate suicidal behavior as a dysfunctional coping strategy. However, as psychiatric disorders and suicidal behavior could share some underlying stressors, it is still unclear whether the stress-diathesis model could explain suicidality itself or rather the predisposition to a psychiatric disorder that could predict suicidality. According to the stress-diathesis model, high levels of impulsiveness, aggression, and hopelessness would represent the core of suicidality. Despite evidence showing that impulsive aggressiveness and hopelessness are among risk factors for suicide attempts, for example, in mood disorder patients [42], there is still debate about the actual role played by emotions and temperament features on suicidal behavior. Even though feelings of hopelessness, emptiness, hostility, impulsiveness, aggressiveness, and anger could indicate a higher risk of suicidality, their correlation is still unclear [5].

Most studies available about the topic of personality traits and suicidal behavior refer to psychobiological models of personality using mainly the following instruments: Temperament and Character Inventory (TCI) [43], NEO-Personality Inventory (NEO-PI) [44], Eysenck Personality Questionnaire (EPQ) [45], TEMPS-A [46], Shedler-Westen Assessment Procedure (SWAP) [48], and the BIG FIVE model [47].

8.1.2 Eysenck Personality Questionnaire

Neuroticism and extraversion are the two temperamental traits that are more often associated with suicidal behavior [49]. By neuroticism, it is meant a stable personality trait that induces a predisposition to a breakdown under stressful situations. Extraversion is commonly intended as the predisposition to look for social interaction with other people. As detailed below, studies using this approach to personality are usually consistent in finding a correlation between suicidality and high levels of neuroticism and between suicidality and low levels of extraversion. A group of Indian researchers, using the Eysenck Personality Questionnaire, found high scores in extraversion and low ones in psychoticism in suicide attempters [50]. Subsequent studies confirmed lower scores in extraversion and in neuroticism in suicide attempters [51, 52]. In another study about a population of suicide attempters aged 75 or more, patients scored higher on neuroticism but lower on extraversion compared to general population controls [53]. High levels in neuroticism could suggest a lower ability to cope successfully with negative events and this mechanism among others (over-arousal/emotional dysregulation, poor help-seeking skills) may help to explain an increased risk for suicidal behavior [54, 55].

Another relevant feature associated with suicidal behavior may be the correlation between neuroticism and impulsiveness: as some authors suggested, this interaction could trigger vulnerability to suicidal behavior in crisis situations [51].

8.1.3 Temperament and Character Inventory

The TCI test is a well-known and useful tool to outline personality traits in patients: it is based on a model of personality which includes seven dimensions, divided into temperament and character. Temperament is identified using four dimensions: Novelty Seeking, which expresses the tendency to seek out new stimuli and experiences, to be easily bored, impulsive, and inclined to avoid monotony; Harm Avoidance, which reflects the tendency to avoid aversive experiences; Reward Dependence, which is the tendency to respond markedly to signals of reward, particularly to verbal signals of sentiment, social approval and support; and persistence, which expresses the preservation of resistance to frustration behavior. Character, instead, is identified through the following three dimensions: Self-Directedness, a measure of self-concepts about oneself, self-acceptance, and the ability to direct one's own life according to personal goals and values; Cooperativeness, which encloses self-concepts about others, and the ability to collaborate well with others; and Self-Transcendence, an expression of the relationship between the self and the external world as an including nature, spirituality, and creativity. Using the TCI test, various studies confirmed that suicide attempters display higher scores in Harm Avoidance, and lower scores in Self-Directedness (SD) and Cooperativeness (C), compared to controls [56–60].

Other variables linked with increased suicide attempts, even though with a weaker association, were higher Novelty Seeking and Self-Transcendence. High levels of Harm Avoidance could be related to dysfunctional and maladaptive coping skills that aim to avoid stressors rather than dealing with them; this approach, in addition to high impulsivity levels seen in Novelty Seeking subjects, could elicitate self-harm and suicide [61].

8.1.4 TEMPS-A

From the perspective of the affective temperament theory, a recent review [62] focused on the possible associations between particular temperaments and suicidal behaviors. Affective temperaments are known as stable individual differences in the expression of primary emotions, resulting in variable reactivity, energy levels, and self-regulation, according to Kraepelin's theory. They can be measured in clinical settings with the TEMPS-A [46], a tool with a quick administration time (110 yes/no items—completion time approximately 15 min), reliable and stable over time. Affective temperaments include the following: depressive temperament (e.g., "I always put the blame on me"); hyperthymic temperament (e.g., "I am usually in a good and joyful mood"); cyclothymic temperament (e.g., "I swing between highs and lows"); irritable (e.g., "I am a grumpy person"); anxious temperament (e.g., "I always think that something bad is going to happen") [63].

In a meta-analysis including 23 studies, all supported associations between TEMPS-A scores and a history of suicide attempts, suicidal ideation, or hopelessness (considered as one of the most important predictors of suicidal behavior). In suicidal subjects, TEMPS-A scores were higher as follows: cyclothymic (73.9%) > depressive (65.2%) > anxious (50.0%) > irritable (26.1%). On the other hand, scores for hyperthymic temperament were significantly lower in suicidal subjects. In addition, the strength of the association of an affective temperament and suicide was ranked as follows: depressive > irritable > cyclothymic > anxious. Lastly, an inverse relationship between suicidal status with hyperthymic temperament was found [62]). When discussing these findings, the Authors concluded that depressive temperament is often associated with Axis I mood disorders and that this relationship could explain the association with suicidal thoughts or behaviors through depression, pessimism, and demoralization. Irritable temperament, instead, may trigger the negative and aggressive emotions associated with suicide. Finally, cyclothymic temperaments are associated with emotional instability, marked mood reactivity, and rapid mood changes, often with severe psychological suffering: for these reasons cyclothymic temperament may contribute to raise the risk of suicide [64]. Hypotheses about the protective role of hyperthymic temperament may regard successful coping strategies related to greater energy, drive, and ambition, as well as cognitive and social/interpersonal skills that can, in conclusion, decrease the risk of suicidal behavior. In this meta-analysis [62], it is also relevant that the findings about temperament and suicidality are coherent in non-mood-disordered psychiatric samples, subjects without psychiatric diagnoses, and those diagnosed with unipolar or bipolar mood disorders. This consistency supports the validity of the reported associations and the stability of the temperament assessments across different samples and comorbidities [65].

8.1.5 Shedler-Westen Assessment Procedure

Another model for personality assessment is the one that can be tested with the Shedler-Westen Assessment Procedure (SWAP), which is a unique psychological test for personality assessment and clinical case formulation. Clinicians can rank order 200 test items into categories from nondescriptive to highly descriptive of the patient. Items are scored 0 (not at all characteristic) to 7 (highly characteristic). The diagnostic scale scores are expressed as T-scores (Mean = 50, SD = 10). The score profiles provide: DSM-5 personality disorder diagnoses; personality diagnoses for alternative, empirically-derived personality syndromes; dimensional trait scores. With this method personality diagnoses are structured in four spectrums: Internalizing Spectrum, Externalizing Spectrum, Borderline-Dysregulated Spectrum, Neurotic Style. The internalizing spectrum subsumes four personality disorders: Depressive, Anxious-Avoidant, Dependent-Victimized, and Schizoid-Schizotypal. Individuals with disorders in the internalizing spectrum experience chronic painful emotions, especially depression and anxiety, tend to be emotionally inhibited and socially avoidant, and tend to blame themselves for their difficulties. The externalizing spectrum subsumes three personality disorders: Antisocial-Psychopathic, Paranoid, and Narcissistic. Individuals with disorders in the externalizing spectrum are angry or hostile, self-centered and lacking in empathy, and blame others for their difficulties. Individuals with Borderline-Dysregulated Personalities have impaired ability to regulate their emotions, have unstable perceptions of self and others that lead to intense and chaotic relationships, and are prone to act on impulses, including self-destructive impulses. The neurotic style grouping subsumes two personality syndromes: Obsessional and Hysteric-Histrionic. These syndromes generally do not entail the same level of impairment or dysfunction as the other personality syndromes, and may therefore be considered character styles rather than disorders. Their more extreme variants can, however, constitute personality disorders [66].

A study using this model [67] involved patients who had already attempted suicide in order to outline patterns of thoughts, feeling, motivation, or behavior—personality patterns—that cause stress or dysfunction. The Authors outlined five personality patterns that could describe suicide attempters' traits and features. Here follows a brief description of each of them. The first three are the most frequently associated with suicide. Firstly, the Authors found an Internalizing subtype (the largest group) that showed chronically depressed, anhedonic, and passive personality features. Externalizer patients, instead, were well represented in the Psychopathic subtype, displaying substance abuse problems, criminality, imperviousness to consequences, and lack of remorse. In addition, difficulty with emotion regulation emerged central to one of the subtypes; the Emotionally Dysregulated subtype, seemingly a close relative of BPD, which mixes elements of internalizing spectrum symptoms with externalizing characteristics. This kind of distinction, internalizing vs. externalizing, is also common in other personality classification systems [68].

The other three subtypes described individuals who do not easily fit into the internalizing-externalizing distinction. The Dependent subtype describes individuals who dream about ideal love, idealize relationships, become attached too quickly, and fear rejection. The Hostile-Isolated subtype is about people that normally tend to avoid social relationships, are critical and competitive toward others. The Anxious-Somatizing subtype features a hypochondriacal patient which tends to use mental and medical issues to avoid responsibility, focusing on avoidance coping strategies. Compared with the first three categories described, these last two are the less frequently associated with suicidality.

8.1.6 The Big Five

The "Big five" is one of the most complete models to outline personality traits, which are subdivided into Openness to experience, Conscientiousness, Extraversion, Agreeableness, and Neuroticism (OCEAN). According to this model, Neuroticism characterizes the tendency to experience negative emotions. Typical adjectives describing neuroticism are moody, nervous, and touchy. Extraversion characterizes positive sensation seeking and the quantity and quality of interpersonal relationships. Typical adjectives describing extraversion are sociable, assertive, and energetic. Openness to experience characterizes autonomous thinking and propensity to try new things. Typical adjectives describing openness are inquisitive, philosophical, and innovative. Agreeableness characterizes the quality of interpersonal interactions along a continuum from social antagonism to compassion. Typical adjectives describing agreeableness are kind, considerate, and generous. Lastly, conscientiousness characterizes a sense of duty, persistence, and self-disciplined goal-directed behavior. Typical adjectives describing conscientiousness are organized, responsible, and efficient. To evaluate which type of personality trait is more linked to suicidality, researchers analyzed past suicide risk, present and potential Suicidal Behavior, and the Big Five (OCEAN) personality traits in a large community sample. This study showed a greater suicidal risk for women with high levels of openness and neuroticism, while in men the risk was raised for low levels of conscientiousness and extraversion [69].

These results were also confirmed by another study [70] with the aim to investigate the differences in personality traits, with particular attention to Neuroticism, in a population recruited from different clinical (inpatients and university students) and sociocultural settings (North, center, south Italy, and middle eastern Austria). In the whole sample, the Extraversion trait, intended as warmth, assertiveness, and activity, was negatively associated with Suicidal Ideation, Intensity of Suicidal Ideation, Global Mental Impairment, and all the other dimensions of psychiatric symptoms. In the same way, but with a weaker association, Agreeableness (courtesy, altruism, and compliance), a trait usually displayed and useful to obtain significant interpersonal relationships, was less associated with suicidality. These results are in line with the current literature that shows the protective role of Extraversion and Agreeableness [71]. On the other hand, high levels of Neuroticism (fear, anger, and impulsivity) can be seen as a risk factor for suicidality, but only when they are influenced by the presence of other psychiatric symptoms such as depressed mood. Similar results were found in an adult population, using the NEO-Personality Inventory, as personality traits associated with suicidality include a positive association with Neuroticism and a negative one with Extraversion [72].

8.2 Interpersonal Theory of Suicide

As described at the beginning of this chapter, Borderline Personality Disorder diagnostic criteria, particularly affective and behavioral dysregulation, may confer suicide risk to the individual, even though pathways are not yet clearly understood. Despite the number of studies about associations between BPD diagnostic criteria and suicidal ideation and behavior, few have approached this complex topic using the framework of a theory of suicide.

As already underscored, understanding the underlying mechanisms that inflate suicidal ideation and behaviors in individuals with personality disorders, and particularly Borderline Personality Disorder is necessary to develop appropriate and targeted interventions for this high-risk population. Three factors have been identified by factor analyses of both DSM-III-R and DSM-IV criteria for Borderline Personality Disorder: affective dysregulation, behavioral dysregulation, and disturbed relatedness [73, 74]. Affective dysregulation includes affective instability, inappropriate anger, and frantic efforts to avoid abandonment; behavioral dysregulation is about impulsivity in at least two potentially self-damaging areas, suicidal/self-mutilative behavior; last, disturbed relatedness means unstable interpersonal relationships, chronic feelings of emptiness, stress-related paranoid ideation [73, 74].

While in a variety of populations (e.g., adolescents, psychiatric patients, and individuals with BPD) the role of both affective and behavioral dysregulation as risk factors for suicidal ideation and attempts is acknowledged, issues concerning the disturbed relatedness factor (such as identity problems, chronic feelings of emptiness) are rarely found to be significantly associated with suicide (see [75] for an exception).

Rogers and coworkers [76] attempted to clarify the aforesaid pathways through the lens of the interpersonal theory of suicide. The Authors predicted that the relationship between affective dysregulation and suicidal ideation would be mediated by perceived burdensomeness and thwarted belongingness, and that behavioral dysregulation would be indirectly associated with a history of suicide attempts through the acquired capability for suicide.

Perceived burdensomeness refers to the view that one's existence is a burden to family, friends, and/or society. This potential misperception may eventually produce the idea that "my death will be worth more than my life to family, friends, society, etc." Thwarted belongingness refers to a poor sense of belongingness, as experienced by one who feels alienated from others, not an integral part of a family, circle of friends, or another valued group. Perceived burdensomeness and/or thwarted belongingness may instill a desire for suicide, but are not enough to turn this desire into an actual suicide attempt. For this, a third element should be involved, i.e., the acquired capability for lethal self-injury. Capability for suicide is acquired through repeated fights with self-preservation motives, which eventually instill the capacity to stare down the self-preservation instinct. According to the principles of the opponent-process theory, as the individual is exposed to an affective stimulus, it eventually loses its ability to elicit the original response, while the opposite response is strengthened [77]. According to this theory, acquired capability for suicide is a continuous and dynamic construct building itself through habituation to repeated exposure to painful or fearsome experiences, which lead to a higher tolerance for pain and a sense of fearlessness in the face of death.

Interestingly, self-mutilation behaviors and non-suicidal self-injury which can be found in Borderline Personality Disorder are in themselves aversive, painful, and provocative events. Repeated exposure to self-harm may lead to a decrease of the original response of fear and pain and increase a response characterized by relief and pain tolerance [78, 79], possibly resulting in increased capability for suicide [80]; furthermore, previous suicide attempts may increase fearlessness about death and pain tolerance, and eventually one's capability to make a lethal suicide attempt [78, 79, 81, 82].

In their study, Rogers and coworkers [76] involved 169 individuals (62.7% female; mean age 26.05, SD = 10.08) seeking outpatient services at a university-based psychological clinic. Findings revealed that the relationship between affective dysregulation and suicidal ideation was fully accounted for by perceived burdensomeness, whereas thwarted belongingness did not explain these associations. Furthermore, the acquired capability for suicide did not explain the association between behavioral dysregulation and suicide attempt history. Thus, it seems that those with dysregulated emotions may experience an internalized sense of being a burden on others, and develop suicidal thoughts as a consequence of that.

A study has investigated the independent relationships between psychopathy, narcissism, and suicidality from the perspective of the interpersonal theory of suicide [83], but results partially supported the study hypotheses. These were about the fact that the impulsive-antisocial facets of psychopathy would be related to suicidal desire, all facets of psychopathy would relate to the capability for suicide; last, that there could be an association between pathological narcissism, thwarted belongingness, and capability for suicide, but not perceived burdensomeness.

According to the framework offered by the interpersonal theory of suicide, it was hypothesized that some mental disorders would better predict suicidal ideation rather than a suicide attempt. This hypothesis was tested in a sample of 997 adult outpatients [84], controlling for sex and age. Thwarted belongingness and perceived burdensomeness were positively associated with those disorders generally symptomatically associated with social withdrawal or potential liability to others (such as depressive and bipolar disorders, social phobia, borderline personality disorder, schizophrenia and other psychotic disorders, drug dependence). On the other hand, it was found an association between acquired capability for suicide and disorders associated with potential exposure to painful and provocative events (such as post-traumatic stress disorder, schizophrenia and other psychotic disorders, drug use).

A study in older people with personality disorder traits supported the role of perceived burdensomeness, thwarted belongingness and depressive symptoms as risk factors for suicidal behaviors [85] and suggested the importance of assessing and addressing the correlates of the interpersonal theory of suicide also in the elderly population.

8.3 Conclusions

Addressing suicide and overall suicidal behaviors in personality disorders is important, considering that they may represent a risk factor for such behaviors. Furthermore, personality organization and personality features, including temperament and character traits, should be addressed as well. Although treatment approaches have been suggested to address suicidality in personality disorders, such as dialectical behavior therapy, mentalization-based therapy, abandonment psychotherapy, and Systems Training for Emotional Predictability and Problem Solving [86–90], further research in this field is still warranted.

Overall, personality disorder patients and those displaying specific personality features which confer them a higher risk for suicidal behavior represent a hard challenge for clinicians and therapists, especially in those cases, like borderline personality disorder, where self-harm behaviors and suicidality are intrinsic features of the individual.

Author Contributions MS and PZ were responsible for the conception of the work; they drafted and revised it critically for important intellectual contents. All authors provided approval for publication of the content.

Conflict of Interest Statement The authors declare that the research was conducted in the absence of any commercial or financial relationships that could be construed as a potential conflict of interest.

References

1. American Psychiatric Association. Diagnostic and statistical manual of mental disorders. 5th ed; 2013. https://doi.org/10.1176/appi.books.9780890425596.
2. Esbec E, Echeburùa E. New criteria for personality disorders in DSM-V. Actas Esp Psiquiatr. 2011;39(1):1–11.
3. Turecki G, Brent D. Suicide and suicidal behavior. Lancet. 2016;387(10024):1227–39. https://doi.org/10.1016/S0140-6736(15)00234-2.
4. CDC. Homicides and suicides—National Violent Death Reporting System. Morb Mortal Wkly Rep. 2006;55:721–4.
5. Giner L, Blasco-Fontecilla H, De La Vega D, Courtet P. Cognitive, emotional, temperament, and personality trait correlates of suicidal behavior. Curr Psychiatry Rep. 2016;18(11):102. https://doi.org/10.1007/s11920-016-0742-x.

6. Pompili M, Ruberto A, Girardi P, Tatarelli R. Suicidality in DSM-IV cluster B personality disorders: an overview. Ann Ist Super Sanita. 2004;40:475–83.
7. Borges G, Nock MK, Haro Abad JM, et al. Twelve-month prevalence of and risk factors for suicide attempts in the World Health Organization World Mental Health Surveys. J Clin Psychiatry. 2010;71(12):1617–28.
8. Halicka J, Kiejna A. Non-suicidal self-injury (NSSI) and suicidal: criteria differentiation. Adv Clin Exp Med. 2018;27(2):257–61. https://doi.org/10.17219/acem/66353.
9. Nock MK, Green JG, Hwang I, et al. Prevalence, correlates, and treatment of lifetime suicidal behavior among adolescents: results from the National Comorbidity Survey Replication Adolescent Supplement. JAMA Psychiatry. 2013;70(3):300–10.
10. Wolff JC, Thompson E, Thomas SA, Nesi J, Bettis AH, Ransford B, Scopelliti K, Frazier EA, Liu RT. Emotion dysregulation and non-suicidal self-injury: a systematic review and meta-analysis. Eur Psychiatry. 2019;59:25–36. https://doi.org/10.1016/j.eurpsy.2019.03.004.
11. World Health Organization. Suicide in the world: global health estimates. World Health Organization. 2009. https://apps.who.int/iris/handle/10665/326948. License: CC BY-NC-SA 3.0 IGO.
12. GBD 2017 Causes of Death Collaborators. Global, regional, and national age-sex-specific mortality for 282 causes of death in 195 countries and territories, 1980-2017: a systematic analysis for the Global Burden of Disease Study 2017. Lancet. 2018;392(10159):1736–88. https://doi.org/10.1016/S0140-6736(18)32203-7.
13. CDC (Centers for Disease Control and Prevention). Definitions: self-directed violence. Atlanta, GA: CDC; 2015. http://www.cdc.gov/violenceprevention/suicide/definitions.html
14. Bachmann S. Epidemiology of suicide and the psychiatric perspective. Int J Environ Res Public Health. 2018;15(7):1425. https://doi.org/10.3390/ijerph15071425.
15. Bertolote JM, Fleischmann A, De Leo D, Wasserman D. Psychiatric diagnoses and suicide: revisiting the evidence. Crisis. 2004;25:147–55. https://doi.org/10.1027/0227-5910.25.4.147.
16. Owens D, House A. General hospital services for deliberate selfharm. Haphazard clinical provision, little research, no central strategy. J R Coll Physicians Lond. 1994;28(4):370–1.
17. Baus N, Fischer-Kern M, Naderer A, Klein J, Doering S, Pastner B, et al. Personality organization in borderline patients with a history of suicide attempts. Psychiatry Res. 2014;218(1–2):129–33. https://doi.org/10.1016/j.psychres.2014.03.048.
18. Ogrodniczuk JS, Piper WE, Joyce AS, Steinberg PI, Duggal S. Interpersonal problems associated with narcissism among psychiatric outpatients. J Psychiatr Res. 2009;43(9):837–42. https://doi.org/10.1016/j.jpsychires.2008.12.005).
19. Doyle M, While D, Mok PL, Windfuhr K, Ashcroft DM, Kontopantelis E, Chew-Graham CA, Appleby L, Shaw J, Webb RT. Suicide risk in primary care patients diagnosed with a personality disorder: a nested case control study. BMC Fam Pract. 2016;17:106. https://doi.org/10.1186/s12875-016-0479-y.
20. Giner L, Blasco-Fontecilla H, Mercedes Perez-Rodriguez M, Garcia-Nieto R, Giner J, Guija JA, Rico A, Barrero E, Luna MA, de Leon J, Oquendo MA, Baca-Garcia E. Personality disorders and health problems distinguish suicide attempters from completers in a direct comparison. J Affect Disord. 2013;151(2):474–83. https://doi.org/10.1016/j.jad.2013.06.029.
21. McGlashan TH. The Chestnut Lodge follow-up study. III. Long term outcome of borderline personalities. Arch Gen Psychiatry. 1986;43:20–30.
22. Stone MH, Stone DK, Hurt SW. Natural history of borderline patients treated by intensive hospitalization. Psychiatr Clin North Am. 1987;10:185–206.
23. Kullgren G, Renberg E, Jacobsson L. An empirical study of borderline personality disorder and psychiatric suicides. J Nerv Ment Dis. 1986;174:328–31.
24. Runeson B, Beskow J. Borderline personality disorder in young Swedish suicides. J Nerv Ment Dis. 1991;179:153–6.
25. Apter A, Bleich A, King RA, Kron S, Fluch A, Kotler M, Cohen DJ. Death without warning? A clinical postmortem study of suicide in 43 Israeli adolescent males. Arch Gen Psychiatry. 1993;50:138–42.

26. Levi-Belz Y, Gvion Y, Levi U, Apter A. Beyond the mental pain: a case-control study on the contribution of schizoid personality disorder symptoms to medically serious suicide attempts. Compr Psychiatry. 2019;90:102–9. https://doi.org/10.1016/j.comppsych.2019.02.005.
27. Stone MH. Long-term follow-up of narcissistic/borderline patients. Psychiatr Clin North Am. 1989;12:621–41.
28. Blasco-Fontecilla H, Baca-Garcia E, Dervic K, Perez-Rodriguez MM, Lopez-Castroman J, Saiz-Ruiz J, Oquendo MA. Specific features of suicidal behavior in patients with narcissistic personality disorder. J Clin Psychiatry. 2009;70(11):1583–7. https://doi.org/10.4088/JCP.08m04899.
29. Garvey MJ, Spoden F. Suicide attempts in antisocial personality disorder. Compr Psychiatry. 1980;21:146–9.
30. Links PS, Heslegrave RJ, Mitton JE, van Reekum R, Patrick J. Borderline personality disorder and substance abuse: consequences of comorbidity. Can J Psychiatr. 1995;40:9–14.
31. Amore M, Innamorati M, Vittorio CD, Weinberg I, Turecki G, Sher L, Paris J, Girardi P, Pompili M. Suicide attempts in major depressed patients with personality disorder. Suicide Life Threat Behav. 2014;44(2):155–66. https://doi.org/10.1111/sltb.12059.
32. Soloff PH, Lis JA, Kelly T, Cornelius J, Ulrich R. Risk factors for suicidal behavior in borderline personality disorder. Am J Psychiatry. 1994;151:1316–23.
33. Lesage AD, Boyer R, Grunberg F, Vanier C, Morissette R, Menard-Buteau C, Loyer M. Suicide and mental disorders: a case-control study of young men. Am J Psychiatry. 1994;151:1063–8.
34. Wedig MM, Silverman MH, Frankenburg FR, Reich DB, Fitzmaurice G, Zanarini MC. Predictors of suicide attempts in patients with borderline personality disorder over 16 years of prospective follow-up. Psychol Med. 2012;42(11):2395–404. https://doi.org/10.1017/S0033291712000517.
35. Brent DA, Johnson BA, Perper J, Connolly J, Bridge J, Bartle S, Rather C. Personality disorder, personality traits, impulsive violence, and completed suicide in adolescents. J Am Acad Child Adolesc Psychiatry. 1994;33(8):1080–6. https://doi.org/10.1097/00004583-199410000-00003.
36. Chioqueta AP, Stiles TC. Assessing suicide risk in cluster C personality disorders. Crisis. 2004;25(3):128–33. https://doi.org/10.1027/0227-5910.25.3.128.
37. Wasserman D, Rihmer Z, Rujescu D, Sarchiapone M, Sokolowski M, Titelman D, Zalsman G, Zemishlany Z, Carli V, European Psychiatric Association. The European Psychiatric Association (EPA) guidance on suicide treatment and prevention. Eur Psychiatry. 2012;27(2):129–41. https://doi.org/10.1016/j.eurpsy.2011.06.003.
38. Ghinea D, Koenig J, Parzer P, Brunner R, Carli V, Hoven CW, Sarchiapone M, Wasserman D, Resch F, Kaess M. Longitudinal development of risk-taking and self-injurious behavior in association with late adolescent borderline personality disorder symptoms. Psychiatry Res. 2019;273:127–33. https://doi.org/10.1016/j.psychres.2019.01.010.
39. Koenig J, Brunner R, Fischer-Waldschmidt G, Parzer P, Plener PL, Park J, Wasserman C, Carli V, Hoven CW, Sarchiapone M, Wasserman D, Resch F, Kaess M. Prospective risk for suicidal thoughts and behaviour in adolescents with onset, maintenance or cessation of direct self-injurious behaviour. Eur Child Adolesc Psychiatry. 2017;26(3):345. https://doi.org/10.1007/s00787-016-0896-4.
40. Nakar O, Brunner R, Schilling O, Chanen A, Fischer G, Parzer P, Carli V, Wasserman D, Sarchiapone M, Wasserman C, Hoven CW, Resch F, Kaess M. Developmental trajectories of self-injurious behavior, suicidal behavior and substance misuse and their association with adolescent borderline personality pathology. J Affect Disord. 2016;197:231–8. https://doi.org/10.1016/j.jad.2016.03.029.
41. Sarchiapone M, Jaussent I, Roy A, Carli V, Guillaume S, Jollant F, Malafosse A, Courtet P. Childhood trauma as a correlative factor of suicidal behavior—via aggression traits. Similar results in an Italian and in a French sample. Eur Psychiatry. 2009;24(1):57–62. https://doi.org/10.1016/j.eurpsy.2008.07.005.
42. Isometsa E. Suicidal behaviour in mood disorders—who, when, and why? Can J Psychiatr. 2014;59(3):120–30.

43. Cloninger C, Przybeck T, Svrakic D, Wetzel R. The Temperament and Character Inventory (TCI): a guide to ITS development and use center for psychobiology of personality. St. Louis: Washington University; 1994.
44. Costa P, McCrae R. Revised NEO personality inventory and NEO five factor inventory professional manual. Odessa: Psychological Assessment Resources; 1992.
45. Eysenck H, Eysenck S. Manual of the Eysenck personality inventory. London: University Press; 1964.
46. Akiskal HS, Akiskal KK, Haykal RF, Manning JS, Connor PD. TEMPS-A: progress towards validation of a self-rated clinical version of the temperament evaluation of the Memphis, Pisa, Paris, and San Diego auto questionnaire. J Affect Disord. 2005;85:3–16.
47. McCrae RR, Costa PT Jr. Validation of the five-factor model of personality across instruments and observers. J Pers Soc Psychol. 1987;52(1):81–90. https://doi.org/10.1037//0022-3514.52.1.81. PMID: 3820081.
48. Shedler J, Westen D. The Shedler-Westen Assessment Procedure (SWAP): making personality diagnosis clinically meaningful. J Pers Assess. 2007;89:41–55.
49. Useda JD, Duberstein PR, Conner KR, Conwell Y. Personality and attempted suicide in depressed adults 50 years of age and older: a facet level analysis. Compr Psychiatry. 2004;45(5):353–61. https://doi.org/10.1016/j.comppsych.2004.06.002.
50. Ponnudurai R, Jeyakar J, Saraswathy M. Attempted suicides in Madras. Indian J Psychiatry. 1986;28(1):59–62.
51. Kumar PN, Rajmohan V, Sushil K. An exploratory analysis of personality factors contributed to suicide attempts. Indian J Psychol Med. 2013;35(4):378–84. https://doi.org/10.4103/0253-7176.122231.
52. Rozanov VA, Mid'ko AA. Personality patterns of suicide attempters: gender differences in Ukraine. Span J Psychol. 2011;14(2):693–700.
53. Wiktorsson S, Berg AI, Billstedt E, Duberstein PR, Marlow T, Skoog I, et al. Neuroticism and extroversion in suicide attempters aged 75 and above and a general population comparison group. Aging Ment Health. 2013;17(4):479–88. https://doi.org/10.1080/13607863.2012.749835.
54. Duberstein PR. Openness to experience and completed suicide across the second half of life. Int Psychogeriatr. 1995;7:183–98.
55. Fergusson DM, Woodward LJ, Horwood LJ. Risk factors and life processes associated with the onset of suicidal behaviour during adolescence and early adulthood. Psychol Med. 2000;30:23–39.
56. Becerra B, Paez F, Robles-Garcia R, Vela GE. Temperament and character profile of persons with suicide attempt. Actas Esp Psiquiatr. 2005;33(2):117–22.
57. Calati R, Giegling I, Rujescu D, Hartmann AM, Moller HJ, De Ronchi D, et al. Temperament and character of suicide attempters. J Psychiatr Res. 2008;42(11):938–45. https://doi.org/10.1016/j.jpsychires.2007.10.006.
58. Ghanem M, Gamaluddin H, Mansour M, Samiee AA, Shaker NM, El Rafei H. Role of impulsivity and other personality dimensions in attempted suicide with self-poisoning among children and adolescents. Arch Suicide Res. 2013;17(3):262–74. https://doi.org/10.1080/13811118.2013.805645.
59. Giegling I, Olgiati P, Hartmann AM, Calati R, Moller HJ, Rujescu D, et al. Personality and attempted suicide. Analysis of anger, aggression and impulsivity. J Psychiatr Res. 2009;43(16):1262–71. https://doi.org/10.1016/j.jpsychires.2009.04.013.
60. Perroud N, Baud P, Ardu S, Krejci I, Mouthon D, Vessaz M, et al. Temperament personality profiles in suicidal behaviour: an investigation of associated demographic, clinical and genetic factors. J Affect Disord. 2013;146(2):246–53. https://doi.org/10.1016/j.jad.2012.09.012.
61. Engstrom C, Brandstrom S, Sigvardsson S, Cloninger CR, Nylander PO. Bipolar disorder. III: harm avoidance a risk factor for suicide attempts. Bipolar Disord. 2004;6(2):130–8.
62. Vázquez GH, et al. Suicidal risk and affective temperaments, evaluated with the temps-a scale: a systematic review. Harv Rev Psychiatry. 2018;26(1):8–18.

63. Rihmer Z, Akiskal KK, Rihmer A, Akiskal HS. Current research on affective temperaments. Curr Opin Psychiatry. 2010;23:12–8.
64. MacKinnon DF, Potash JB, McMahon FJ, et al. Rapid mood switching and suicidality in familial bipolar disorder. Bipolar Disord. 2005;7:441–8.
65. Pompili M, Rihmer Z, Akiskal HS, Innamorati M, Iliceto P, Akiskal KK, Lester D, Narciso V, Ferracuti S, Tatarelli R, De Pisa E, Girardi P. Temperament and personality dimensions in suicidal and nonsuicidal psychiatric inpatients. Psychopathology. 2008;41(5):313–21. https://doi.org/10.1159/000146069. Epub 2008 Jul 19. PMID: 18635934.
66. Westen D, et al. An empirically derived taxonomy for personality diagnosis: bridging science and practice in conceptualizing personality. Am J Psychiatry. 2012;169:273–84.
67. Kile M, et al. Personality subtypes of suicidal adults. J Nerv Ment Dis. 2009;197(9):687–94. https://doi.org/10.1097/NMD.0b013e3181b3b13f.
68. Krueger RF, Tackett JL, editors. Personality and psychopathology. New York, NY: Guilford Press; 2006.
69. Bluml V, Kapusta ND, Doering S, Brahler E, Wagner B, Kerstin A. Personality factors and suicide risk in a representative sample of the German general population. PLoS One. 2013;8:e76646.
70. Stefa-Missagli S, et al. Suicide and personality traits: a multicenter study of Austrian and Italian psychiatric patients and students. Suicide Life Threat Behav. 2019;50(1):220–32. https://doi.org/10.1111/sltb.12579.
71. McCann SJ. Suicide, big five personality factors, and depression at the American state level. Arch Suicide Res. 2010;14:368–74.
72. Chioqueta AP, Stiles TC. Personality traits and the development of depression, hopelessness, and suicide ideation. Personal Individ Differ. 2005;38:1283–91.
73. Sanislow CA, Grilo CM, McGlashan TH. Factor analysis of the DSM-III-R borderline personality disorder criteria in psychiatric inpatients. Am J Psychiatry. 2000;157:1629–33. https://doi.org/10.1176/appi.ajp.157.10.1629.
74. Sanislow CA, Grilo CM, Morey LC, Bender DS, Skodol AE, Gunderson JG, McGlashan TH. Confirmatory factor analysis of DSM-IV criteria for borderline personality disorder: findings from the collaborative longitudinal personality disorders study. Am J Psychiatry. 2002;159:284–90. https://doi.org/10.1176/appi.ajp.159.2.284.
75. Allen B, Cramer RJ, Harris PB, Rufino KA. Borderline personality symptomatology as a mediator of the link between child maltreatment and adult suicide potential. Arch Suicide Res. 2013;17:41–51. https://doi.org/10.1080/13811118.2013.748413.
76. Rogers ML, Joiner TE Jr. Borderline personality disorder diagnostic criteria as risk factors for suicidal behavior through the lens of the interpersonal theory of suicide. Arch Suicide Res. 2016;20(4):591–604. https://doi.org/10.1080/13811118.2016.1158681.
77. Solomon RL. The opponent-process theory of acquired motivation: the costs of pleasure and benefits of pain. Am Psychol. 1980;35:691–712.
78. Joiner TE. Why people die by suicide. Cambridge, MA: Harvard University Press; 2005.
79. Van Orden KA, Witte TK, Cukrowicz KC, Braithwaite SR, Selby EA, Joiner TEJ. The interpersonal theory of suicide. Psychol Rev. 2010;117:575–600. https://doi.org/10.1037/a0018697.
80. Franklin JC, Hessel ET, Prinstein MJ. Clarifying the role of pain tolerance in suicidal capability. Psychiatry Res. 2011;189:362–7. https://doi.org/10.1016/j.psychres.2011.08.001.
81. Anestis MD, Soberay KA, Gutierrez PM, Hernández TD, Joiner TE. Reconsidering the link between impulsivity and suicidal behavior. Personal Soc Psychol Rev. 2014;18:366–86. https://doi.org/10.1177/1088868314535988.
82. Smith PN, Cukrowicz KC, Poindexter EK, Hobson V, Cohen LM. The acquired capability for suicide: a comparison of suicide attempters, suicide ideators, and non-suicidal controls. Depress Anxiety. 2010;27:871–7. https://doi.org/10.1002/da.20701.
83. Harrop TM, Preston OC, Khazem LR, Anestis MD, Junearick R, Green BA, Anestis JC. Dark traits and suicide: associations between psychopathy, narcissism, and components of the interpersonal-psychological theory of suicide. J Abnorm Psychol. 2017;126(7):928–38. https://doi.org/10.1037/abn0000300.

84. Silva C, Ribeiro JD, Joiner TE. Mental disorders and thwarted belongingness, perceived burdensomeness, and acquired capability for suicide. Psychiatry Res. 2015;226(1):316–27. https://doi.org/10.1016/j.psychres.2015.01.008.
85. Jahn DR, Poindexter EK, Cukrowicz KC. Personality disorder traits, risk factors, and suicide ideation among older adults. Int Psychogeriatr. 2015;27(11):1785–94. https://doi.org/10.1017/S1041610215000174.
86. Andreoli A, Burnand Y, Cochennec MF, Ohlendorf P, Frambati L, Gaudry-Maire D, Di Clemente T, Hourton G, Lorillard S, Canuto A, Frances A. Disappointed love and suicide: a randomized controlled trial of "abandonment psychotherapy" among borderline patients. J Personal Disord. 2016;30(2):271–87. https://doi.org/10.1521/pedi_2015_29_196.
87. Bateman A, Fonagy P. Effectiveness of partial hospitalization in the treatment of borderline personality disorder: a randomized controlled trial. Am J Psychiatry. 1999;156(10):1563–9. https://doi.org/10.1176/ajp.156.10.1563.
88. Bateman A, Fonagy P. 8-year follow-up of patients treated for borderline personality disorder: mentalization-based treatment versus treatment as usual. Am J Psychiatry. 2008;165(5):631–8. https://doi.org/10.1176/appi.ajp.2007.07040636.
89. Boccalon S, Alesiani R, Giarolli L, Fossati A. Systems training for emotional predictability and problem solving program and emotion dysregulation: a pilot study. J Nerv Ment Dis. 2017;205(3):213–6. https://doi.org/10.1097/NMD.0000000000000640.
90. Linehan MM, Comtois KA, Murray AM, Brown MZ, Gallop RJ, Heard HL, Korslund KE, Tutek DA, Reynolds SK, Lindenboim N. Two-year randomized controlled trial and follow-up of dialectical behavior therapy vs therapy by experts for suicidal behaviors and borderline personality disorder. Arch Gen Psychiatry. 2006;63(7):757–66. https://doi.org/10.1001/archpsyc.63.7.757. Erratum in: ArchGen Psychiatry. 2007 Dec;64(12):1401

MIX
Papier aus verantwortungsvollen Quellen
Paper from responsible sources
FSC® C105338

If you have any concerns about our products,
you can contact us on
ProductSafety@springernature.com

In case Publisher is established outside the EU,
the EU authorized representative is:
Springer Nature Customer Service Center GmbH
Europaplatz 3, 69115 Heidelberg, Germany

Printed by Libri Plureos GmbH
in Hamburg, Germany